SHAKE YOUR HEAD, DARLING

SHAKE YOUR HEAD, DARLING

by Jose Eber

Photographs by Steve Schapiro

WARNER BOOKS

A Warner Communications Company

Photographs of Cher by Harry Langdon
Makeup by James Cooper Jr.

An excerpt from this book first appeared in *Ladies' Home Journal.*

Warner Books, Inc., 666 Fifth Avenue, New York, N.Y. 10103

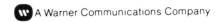 A Warner Communications Company

Printed in the United States of America
First printing: February 1983
10 9 8 7 6 5 4 3 2

Library of Congress Cataloging in Publication Data

Eber, Jose.
  Shake your head, darling.

  1. Hairdressing. I. Title.
TT972.E185   1983   646.7′24   82-50639
ISBN 0-446-51250-8   AACR2

Book design: H. Roberts Design

To my mother, who has believed in me all my life, especially from the time I was twelve years old and wanted to be a little bit different. She has always accepted me, eccentricities and all, and never criticized me. She encouraged me to be me, and stood up to my father, who, in the early years, was very much against my being a hairstylist. To my father, who, even though he did not see my future as I did, would be proud of what I have accomplished. To my sister, Esther, and my brother, Henri, who have helped to keep our family close.

Contents

Acknowledgments

There are many people I would like to thank for their help in making this book possible: Maurice Azoulay, my partner, who had to deal with my absence from the shop to work on this book; Blake Ballard; Henri Belolo, for his kindness and support; Executive Producer Marty Berman, Karen Cadle, Steve Clements, and Gary Collins from *Hour Magazine* and the staff, who is so patient; James Cooper, J. C., who did the makeup in this book and who gives the finishing touch, a perfect makeup, to each of the photographs and is a wonderful friend; Joel Gotler, my agent (I don't do his hair); George Kirvay and Alan Neirob, my publicists, who help with all things; Sonia Leb, who had stood by my side for the past six years and who helps me always; Jacques Morali, who is in part responsible for my coming to America, and whose friendship I highly regard; Nansey Neiman and Howard Kaminsky, of Warner Books, Inc., who believed in me from the start and helped me to bring this book to you; Marge Schicktanz, for her time and effort; Louis Torres, who has been a great friend over the years; and at the shop, Araxy Besnelian, my colorist, who adds an extra sparkle to the hair of many of my clients, Irene Zito, and Janet Leigh; and Steve West, for his assistance throughout the making of this book. And special thanks to Fran Curtis and Edna Farley.

I also want to thank Steve Schapiro, Maura Smith, and Louis A. Schaffner, and Suzy Kalter, my collaborator, without whom I could not have written this. She has become part of my family.

Part One:

THE FACTS

Shake your head, darling. That's right, put this book down and let loose. Roll your neck from side to side and let your hair fly.

That's what I thought. Dull. Listless. No oomph. Hasn't got the kind of sparkle you've been dreaming of, hm? I know. I see it every day—hundreds of women not looking as good as they should, simply because their hair hasn't got real pizzaz. Let's face it. You deserve to look better.

That's why I'm here. By the time we're finished, you'll be a prettier you. When you shake your head, the world will applaud. I know, because I've already helped thousands of women just like you.

My name is Jose Eber. That's Joe-zey, darling, not Hoe-say, because I'm French. I'm a hairstylist in Beverly Hills, where I own a salon, one block from Rodeo Drive, called Maurice/Jose. You've heard of it? I hope so. Our clientele includes many celebrities, recording stars, television stars, movie stars, and all that . . . and thousands of working women, who come to us not because we do the stars but because we are life-style experts.

I was born in Nice, in the south of France. I wanted to go into show business until one magic day when I was thirteen. Then I started cutting my sister and my mother's hair—no training, no nothing. They were very brave. At least, I think so. I just had an urge to do it, and it turned out that I had a natural talent for hair. My hands had the feel, or however you call it. They knew what to do. My family moved to Germany when I was fifteen, and I got my first job, at the beauty parlor in the Berlin Hilton Hotel. That was the first time I met Americans, and from the beginning I loved them. From Berlin I moved to Paris, where they were not sitting around waiting for me, believe me. I had to work very hard, but this was what I wanted, and so I became the number-one scissors at a big, fancy salon in Paris. But when I went to the U.S. on holiday, I fell in love with Los Angeles and decided to start my life over, American style. So I sold all my belongings, everything, and took a job in Beverly Hills. Soon the models and the celebrities started to come to me: Susie Coehlo, Farrah Fawcett, Ali MacGraw, Cher, Victoria Principal, Linda Gray, Angie Dickinson, Barbara Walters—everyone I could ever have dreamed of.

Of course, not everyone who comes to me is a movie star; I have about two million clients I have never even met! They watch me on *Hour Magazine*, on the television set. I'm not all glitz and glamour, though. Besides the celebrities and the television show, I work with hundreds of real-live, regular women every week. They come to

1

me for advice. I cut their hair, we talk about permanents, about hair care, about their life-styles, and I give them a new way to be free—free to look their best with a minimum of care. And that's what this book is all about. What goes on between me and a client in my salon is what you are going to experience by reading this book.

There are many, many beauty books on the market, and they all have pretty much one thing in common: they tell you to pick the best hairstyle for your face, without ever taking your life-style into consideration. They assume that looking best is a problem you can easily overcome once you know what hairstyle looks right with your face shape. I say this is all true—yes, it is very good advice—but the hairstyle is useless if you can't do it yourself and it doesn't fit into your time schedule. Darling, I don't care how gorgeous you look in a certain style; if you haven't got time for the electric rollers or whatever else it takes to get that look for you, then it's simply not right. And you shouldn't think twice about it.

Face shape is important, but life-style is more important. I say, you are you. This is the first beauty book that is written to show you how to come up with the right options for all the variables in your beauty life, including your life-style, your face shape, your hair type, and your age. When you are finished with this book, it will be as if I have stepped out of its pages and into your home or your bathroom with you—it's okay, I do some of my best work in bathrooms. It will be just as if you had had an in-person consultation in my salon, in Beverly Hills. If you use this as a workbook, you'll save yourself the price of a plane ticket to Los Angeles and the $100 I charge for a haircut. The results will be almost the same, and you won't have jet lag.

I think women today have many opportunities to do whatever they want, and that individual hairstyles have a new status; the single "fashion" hairstyle is less important. No longer can a movie star or a President's wife dictate the "in" way to wear your hair. Women will no longer torture themselves to have a single style that is "in" rather than one that may look better or is easier for them but is "out." Life-style and convenience have, by necessity, merged, and the woman of today can look fashionable and still choose a hairstyle and beauty plan that is tailor-made for her personal way of life.

If you are a working woman or a mother and have only a few minutes in the morning for your daily beauty rituals, you must have a hairstyle that reacts perfectly, or you are going to be angry, frustrated, ugly, or all three. And we don't want that, do we?

There are some women who have nothing to do in the morning but take care of themselves. I think that's terrific. These women invariably look divine. Electric rollers, intricate hairstyles, and elaborate plans are fine for them. Their hours in front of the mirror pay off when they finally emerge, triumphantly beautiful. Other women have a total of about twenty or thirty minutes each morning in which to shower, dress, fix their hair, and apply their makeup—and they may not get a chance even to perform a touch-up later on in the day. These women need a look that they can fix once and will last them until bedtime. There are other women who really mean to set time aside each day for hair and beauty but, because they have small children or a household emergency or errands to do or they're involved in sports, they just never get around to spending any time on themselves. Or maybe they have a quick five minutes, and their hope is that someday, someone will invent a way for them to wake up looking perfect, so they can save the five minutes.

All of these types of women have completely different life-styles, so the shape of their face is secondary in choosing the right hairstyle. Among my clients, I see that there are really three basic life-styles: sporty, working woman, and nonworking woman. I call these Red, Green, and Blue, so I have divided this book into these three categories to help you find the hairstyles that are you.

We all know life is not so simple that you will fall into a neat category. But time after time, I see women with the same kinds of problems, and they more or less break down the same way. So take my Life-style Quiz and see where you end up. I'm not saying this is a perfect science. In the shop, I would see you in front of me. But since this is a book, you must help me to see you better.

These are the questions I would ask of you if you came into my shop. In person I would touch your hair, I would ask you to shake your head, I would see the way you walk and hear the way you talk. I'd see how you take your coffee and what kind of magazines you read while you're waiting for a shampoo. All these things matter in choosing a hairstyle. So give me a hand. Let's work together, and together we'll make being a more beautiful you a simple task.

Just answer these questions.

JOSE EBER'S LIFE-STYLE QUIZ

1. **When I wake up in the morning:**
   A. I look at the alarm clock and panic. I'm already late.
   B. Who needs an alarm clock? I'm up with the birds, or the kids, and ready to go.
   C. I roll over and go back to sleep for another half hour.

2. **My regular morning routine:**
   A. Takes no more than half an hour, total.
   B. Is postponed until later in the day, because of kids, errands, or sports.
   C. Depends on what I'm doing during the day and my evening plans.

3. **When I look in the mirror each morning I:**
   A. Wish I had time to do something about what I see.
   B. Splash cold water on my face and check the condition of my skin.
   C. Study each line, blemish, and soft spot mercilessly, until I'm satisfied I know exactly how to best care for what I've seen.

4. **First thing in the morning, my hair:**
   A. Needs a wash and blow-dry to look decent.
   B. Kind of falls into place, because my haircut is easy to care for.
   C. Is almost perfect, because I just had it done yesterday.

5. **My hair:**
   A. Gets cut whenever I'm in the mood or it's reached the unbearable stage.
   B. Needs to be cut every four–six weeks; otherwise it's unmanageable.
   C. Is long, to allow for a variety of styles, so I just get the ends trimmed regularly.

6. **My hair color:**
   A. Is something I've experimented with myself.
   B. Yuck! Ruin my hair with chemicals?
   C. Is done at the beauty shop every four–six weeks.

7. **The colors I most frequently wear are:**
   A. Safe and look smart in the business world: neutrals, navy, burgundy.
   B. Bright colors and "fashion" colors. I love them all.
   C. Whatever the fashion experts say is "in" this year.

8. **For a purse, I usually carry:**
   A. One good all-purpose bag that goes with everything.
   B. Something fun and inexpensive that holds all my junk.
   C. Whatever matches my clothes.

9. **The hair appliances I rely on include:**
   A. A round brush and blow-dryer.
   B. I have all kinds of stuff, but I never use it.
   C. Electric rollers, hairpins, combs, clips, curling iron, crimper, dryers, and brushes.

10. **For breakfast, I:**
    A. Grab something on the way to work or eat at my desk.
    B. Have cold cereal and fruit or something sensible.
    C. Have a light meal, or a little more if I'm eating a late lunch.

11. **When I bathe, I:**
    A. Take a shower first thing in the morning.
    B. Take a shower or a bath several times a day, after sports activities.
    C. Take a leisurely bath.

12. **I have help in my home:**
    A. Never.
    B. Once or twice a week.
    C. Full time.

13. **I put myself together:**
    A. To please myself.
    B. To suit my life-style.
    C. To please my man.

14. **I work:**
    A. At a regular job.
    B. You think taking care of the kids isn't full-time work?
    C. Flexible hours or not at all.

15. **My fingernails:**
    A. Are manicured by me.
    B. Are kept neat and short for simplicity.
    C. Are manicured regularly.

16. **When it comes to athletics:**
    A. Weekends are the only time I have for recreational sports.
    B. I'd only be more active if I were training for the Olympics.
    C. I don't sweat.

17. If I have a little extra money to splurge with, I:
   A. Buy something I need.
   B. Get something for someone else.
   C. Buy something wonderful I'm dying to have but don't really need.

18. My idea of the perfect vacation would be to:
   A. Travel to the major cities of Europe.
   B. Go hiking or backpacking.
   C. Escape to a spa.

19. My bedtime is:
   A. After the 11:00 P.M. news.
   B. I crash early, after an exhausting day.
   C. Whenever the party's over.

20. If I could sum up my beauty routine simply, I would say it's:
   A. Sensible.
   B. Practical.
   C. Time-consuming.

Now let's figure out your score. For each "A" answer, you get two points; for each "B" answer, you get one point; and for each "C" answer, you get three points.

LIFE-STYLE RED

If your score is 20–30, you are a Life-style Red. You have a crazy, busy life-style that either involves children, several sports activities, or a few jobs. You are always running around, with little time to spare for yourself. You need a hairstyle and beauty routine that can withstand lack of attention, several showers, extremes in location— you're in and out of doors constantly, in and out of the car several times during the day, and always, always on the go. You have no time to primp or stop by the ladies' room to check your hairstyle. You care about your body, your health, the food you eat, and the activities you pursue, even though you find that lack of time often works against your best intentions. There are many things you mean to do, but you just don't have time for all of them.

LIFE-STYLE GREEN

If your score is 31–40, you are a Life-style Green. You're a working woman, with or without children. You care about your looks but you have a limited amount of time to commit to beauty rituals. You want to look your best but you can't get involved in any complicated hairstyles. Just finding the time to get to the beauty salon for a trim is difficult for you. You like to know that when you put your face on in the morning and comb your hair, your "look" will last all day and maybe into the evening. You carry lipstick and a refresher kit in your handbag but rarely have time to indulge in a touch-up. You need a non-stop look that gives you the confidence to know, without having constantly to consult a mirror, your appearance is always perfect.

LIFE-STYLE BLUE

If your score is over 40, you are a Life-style Blue. Lucky you—your time is your own, and you are in command of your day and your looks. You have the time, patience, and funds to shop for just the right clothes for your figure; and the time to work with your hair until it's exactly the way you want it. You think nothing of changing your clothes or your hairstyle, even in the same day. Your main desire is to look as good as you can. You're no novice when it comes to coloring, treatments, and the latest in hair accessories. You are the woman every other woman envies.

●‖●‖●‖●‖●

The Life-style Quiz works best for someone with a distinct life-style. Some people had a bit of a overlap into Red or Green and are Blue on special occasions. When I sat down and talked to these people, I found they had a conflict: while they really did fit into a certain life-style, often they did not allow themselves the time to fit into it. Women who worked in an office who basically tested out to be Life-style Green were not giving themselves a full thirty to sixty minutes in the morning for their routine. Yet they were not Life-style Red profiles. If you are cheating on your life-style, darling, that's your business. But don't cheat on me, or I won't be able to help you. If you are a Life-style Green and you want a Life-style Red hairstyle, I can help you, but don't blame me if you haven't got as many choices as you would like. Red hairstyles are for women who are active in sports or who run around with small children all the time and have absolutely no time for themselves. Green hairstyles are for women who work with other people.

So how did you do? Do you want to take the test over again? Be my guest. Then go to the back of the book and find the section for your life-style profile. This profile is not a silly gimmick, and it's very important for you to know that. My entire career has been based on matching the woman with the right hairstyle, and the hairstyle is only right when it matches the life-style. I am making war on the "done" look, the teased, the sprayed, the beauty-parlor look that some people still think is chic. I am fighting the look-alike philosophy that makes millions of people copy something on someone else—and believe me, I know all about this, because Farrah Fawcett has been my client for a long, long time. I do battle with every hairdresser in this country—no, this world—who wants you to look like someone else or his idea of what you should be looking like during this "fashion season."

What I want for you is a flattering hairstyle you can handle yourself, that looks totally natural, and is soft and becoming and sexy. Every woman deserves to be sexy, and there are ways of being sexy without looking inappropriate in terms of your job or your life-style. Wait and see—I will show you before we're done.

The whole idea of beauty is camouflage. No, no, what I mean is that the whole trick to beauty is camouflage, and a woman's—or a man's, for that matter—best material for camouflage is hair. If your hair looks great, it doesn't matter whether you have makeup on or not, whether you are wearing blue jeans and a sweater or a designer original: something about you looks finished, polished, and alluring. No makeup or fancy clothes will change your general appearance. You might just as well walk around town conducting your business with a paper bag over your head.

Now, then, there is a difference between walking out of a beauty shop looking great and waking up in the morning looking great. This difference is usually based on the haircut, but there are other factors involved as well. For instance, some people have good hands for hair—they just do their hair better than other people; some people have hair that's better to work with than others, or easier, if not better; and there are loads of other variables that we will talk about later. All of these can be taken into consideration, so that it is possible to wake up in the morning and, in the time it takes to snap the fingers, *voilà*, have a hairstyle that you love, looks good on you, represents your own personal look, and meets the requirements of your life-style.

I think that true beauty is a combination of many things. It is not perfect beauty, the kind a movie star or a statue has. It is something that comes partly from within you, has a mental or psychological element, and can be done to you by a professional who knows the tricks of optical illusion. You can be *made* to look beautiful even if, bare-faced in front of the mirror each morning, you really are not.

I cannot help you very much to believe in yourself. I *can* make you look your best so that you can see how good you can look. And then you will believe in what you can do to yourself. But I cannot step within your soul to give you the confidence that real beauty needs. That is up to you.

I can, however, turn an old frump into a beauty queen. I can make a middle-aged woman look ten or fifteen years younger. I can make a hard-edged, tough-looking woman turn soft and sexy and vulnerable. Even a shy woman may turn bold. Hair can make you be almost anybody you want—for a night, a few days, months, or a lifetime. You can shed aspects of your old personality by getting a new hairstyle. I've seen women take on a new air of confidence as they left the salon. I've seen them feel they could own the world because they had a brand-new image.

Maybe ten to twenty percent of the women on earth are beautiful to the point of perfection. No matter what happens, these women are always beautiful. For the remaining eighty or ninety percent, half of beauty is properly using what they have, and the other half is pure illusion. And for those who look better than others, it's not that God made them better than their next-door neighbor—it's just that they have learned more tricks.

A lot of beauty is taking the time to look beautiful. And this is where life-style is so important. There are millions of women in this country who have the potential to be as beautiful as any star you see on screen or stage. Maybe they don't know the tricks of illusion or don't take the time to use them. But being beautiful is hard work. And if you want to look that way, then you have to devote time to it. Your beauty look is probably habit with you. You have appeared the same for so long that it's easy to maintain this look—whether it's the right one for you or not. To change your look is like changing an old habit, and it's trouble for you, so you give up or don't try. A good cut is the basis for your beauty, but the time you take to supplement your beauty routine is the fuel that will keep you running and glowing.

Your hairstylist should help you create a style that works as an optical illusion for your face. Your good points should be shown off, and your bad points softened or covered or hidden. And the style must be something you can do yourself in the amount of time you honestly know you will give yourself for a beauty routine. The goal is to create something that you can happily live with and will also make you look your best.

Think of all the times you have been in a restaurant or at a party or a meeting and a woman has walked into the room and you've hated her because she appears so perfect. She floats instead of walks. Her posture shows her self-confidence. Her clothes, her makeup and her hair are *le dernier cri*, the last word. You think she is absolutely beautiful. Then, because you can't stop staring at her, you get a better look. Her nose is too long, her mouth too big, her jaw too wide. She's very ordinary. In fact, you are prettier. So why did she take your breath away? Because her total look was created to give the illusion of perfect beauty. She is in control.

You can be too, darling.

Part Two:

THE VARIABLES

Once you know your life-style score, you are ready to investigate the other variables that will influence the choice of a hairstyle. I've come up with seven different factors that I think need to be taken into consideration before you even consult with a hairdresser, and these seven variables apply to every person in one way or another. There will be aspects of each variable that don't apply to you, so this is where you have to pick and choose the right information. But be sure you hit all seven categories!

Just to make sure you don't miss anything, there's a worksheet to help you see the facts.

If we all had the same-shape face and the same kind of hair, then life would be very easy—boring, but easy.

Hairstyles would long ago have been perfected, and we would all wear them as if they were uniforms. We might just as well be bald! Luckily, each one of us is different, and it's the ability to work with those differences and to use the tricks of optical illusion that we discussed in Part One that allows us to transform ourselves into creatures of style and taste.

FACE SHAPE

Let's face it, darling, your face is yours—and yours alone. Unless you have a twin or a clone, your face is as unique as your fingerprint. So to make a prettier you, we both need a very good understanding of what's on your face.

You doubtless think you know all about your face—after all, it is your face, and you've probably had it for years. But that could be the problem. Many people look at their face constantly but stop seeing themselves as they really are. And once you start to deal with what you think you look like rather than what you really do look like, you begin to make little mistakes that can detract from a prettier you.

So let's get small. Let's start at the beginning and scrutinize your face, your neck, your ears, your features, and the very shape of your face. Having a flattering hairstyle is not solely dependent on the shape of your face. This is a myth, darling. The way the features of your face are put together, to me, are part of what is structurally your face shape. You may have a round face and Valerie Perrine may have a round face, but believe me, the same hairstyle may not look the same on both of you. So let's forget about Valerie Perrine—or whatever other movie star or famous person you think you might resemble—and concentrate on you, and you alone.

There has been a lot written and said about face shape, and I think most of it is garbage. American women have been trained to spend hours poring over little drawings in magazines, trying to figure out if their face shape matches any of the twelve illustrations. Then they decide which of these shapes they have, label it with a fancy name, and go through life saying, "Hey, wait, I can't wear certain styles because I have a heart-shaped diamond face," or something silly like that.

Then, to make it worse, after years of thinking her face is like a heart-shaped diamond, the woman is told by someone else that it's not a heart-shaped diamond at all; it's an inverted pear. Panic sets in. Confusion reigns. Women get confused and then angry, and yet they still buy the principle that there are lots of different face shapes in cute little categories, and the key to their success in beauty is to find the right category for themselves. This is all wrong.

So I'm telling you now: the more facial shapes you read about, the more you are being taken by a twenty-five-year-old gimmick. This is where I have to say: Come on, darling, trust me. You bought this book, didn't you? You know how many clients depend on me. You know I wouldn't lead you astray. Listen to me. All those crazy face shapes are nonsense. There are only three face shapes you need to know: round, oval, and long. Beyond that, all the differences are in structure. And there are so many possible differences in structure that we can't begin to list them all, because, as we've already said, everyone is different. And those structural differences are what make you unique.

I can line up ten women with round faces, and you would see ten completely different-looking women, who should probably wear ten completely different hairstyles. None of the ten of them will look the same when they stand in that line, and none of the ten will look the same when I fix their hair. Face shape works with several other features on the face to present a total face picture.

Here are the variables that we will take into consideration in determining your face picture:

Actual face shape: Round, oval, or long?

Forehead: High? Low? None? Everybody has a forehead.

Eyes: Don't tell me, let me guess—you've got two!

Nose: Big? Small? Long and thin? You don't need plastic surgery. Or maybe you do.

Ears: Do your ears hang down, do they wobble to and fro? If you've got Prince Charles's ears, you certainly don't want to show them off!

Neck: The length of your neck has a lot to do with the proportions of your haircut, so let's not ignore the neck.

Shoulders: I know you've got one on each side, darling; don't get cute with me. Are they wide or narrow? Do they support a long neck or a short neck? Maybe you have no shoulders and no neck, just three chins. This is not very good. You'll need a lot of help!

Mouth: You have to hear this story, darling. I never thought that mouth had that much to do with hairstyle, but Victoria Principal has been telling me that since I cut her hair, more and more people comment on how beautiful her mouth is; before, they never even knew she had a mouth. Amazing, isn't it? But it's the truth.

You know, I'm sure that very few people have perfectly formed faces. The success of the optical illusion is to make the separate pieces you have work all together in one grand beauty scheme so that you appear to be beautiful. Makeup will do some of this for you, but more important than makeup is the proper hairstyle. If you have a round face, the right hairstyle will make your face look thinner. The wrong hairstyle will make it look fatter. You get the general idea.

Now the subject of face shape becomes very simple. I'm only giving you three categories to choose from.

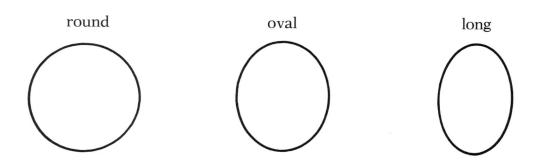

round   oval   long

So go into the bathroom, turn on all the lights, and either pull your hair back into a ponytail or put on a shower cap, so that all you can see is your face and your features. This isn't beauty-contest time, darling, it's honesty time. And it's very important that you be honest, so we can get an accurate idea of what you're going to camouflage. Even if your features are perfect and you are a goddess, let's go in the bathroom and take it from there.

Good. Now wash your face and take a good, hard look at your naked face. Trace the outline of your bone structure with your finger. Learn the distinctions made in the geography of your face by your cheekbones, your jawline, and your actual face shape. Decide now if your face is round, oval, or long. If you always thought you had a triangular face, it's possible that you have an oval face with high protruding cheekbones and a disappearing jawline. Isolate the parts that make up your face. You'll need to know them in a few minutes anyway.

Now, on the worksheet, chronicle each of the features that make up your face picture.

Are your eyes big or small, wide or narrow, set back or set forward? Are they one of your best features or one of your worst? If you don't tell the truth, then how can I help you? Do you wear glasses? If so, don't be embarrassed. Get them out. You should do this analysis with your glasses on.

Eyes: If you have good eyes, then you'll want to accentuate them, maybe with bangs that sweep up and off to one side. If you have great eyes and no forehead, you can still have bangs; just make sure they start way back at the crown, giving the illusion of a high forehead. If you wear glasses, then make sure your bangs aren't too long. If your eyes bulge out of your head, then soften them with softer bangs that frame your face and take away emphasis from your eyes—avoid a heavy bang, which might point to a less-than-perfect feature. Makeup can enhance your eyes, but your hairstyle should frame your eyes as well.

Nose: There is not much a hairstyle can do if you have a really bad nose, but always take one thing into account: keep your hairstyle swept up and away from your face. You don't want any hair covering the lines of your face or drawing more attention to your nose. You want a soft look, a swept-away look. With either long or short hair, it's up and out at the temples to frame your nose. Don't try to hide your nose by having your hair cover your face; that makes everything worse. Consider bangs. Every woman can wear bangs—they frame the eyes and take emphasis away from the nose. If your nose is really huge, hooked, and absolutely terrible, and plastic surgery is out of the question—do what some of the major "beauties" of the world do. Wear an extreme hairstyle and act like you're gorgeous. Think of Diana Vreeland.

Forehead: Do you have a high forehead or a low one? Is it large or small? Do you have a widow's peak? If your forehead is small, bangs can be cut from high on the crown to give the illusion of a larger forehead. If your forehead is large, you must have bangs.

Ears: If your ears stick out like Dumbo's, you don't want to accenuate them. Pull your hair back and take a look at your ears. If they stick out, maybe they should be covered. Avoid geometric and short haircuts. Cover your ears with softness. Flat ears are beautiful, darling; you can show them off.

Mouth: Did you ever look at someone's mouth? Sometimes you don't even think of it. But hair and makeup can emphasize a mouth or do the reverse. A large mouth needs to be balanced by the hair. A small mouth can be corrected with makeup. The mouth should be in tune with the hair: soft, sensuous, touchable.

Jawline: The jawline is one of the most fascinating aspects of face shape, because it changes facial shape. I consider it one of the more basic parts of the face picture. If you have a large jaw, don't try to hide it with hair. That will only accentuate the problem. If you have no jawline, open your face up with upsweep in your hairstyle. Because the jaw is in the lower part of your face picture, use the upper part of the face and the hair that surrounds it to balance the jaw.

Neck: Long neck, short neck? Several chins? Thick neck? Skinny neck? You'll want to show off a long neck, but camouflage one that's too long with lots of soft hair. Yes, darling, a neck can be too long. It's not like being too rich or too thin. A long or short neck needs the right hairstyle and the right clothes. With a tapered hairdo cut close to the head, you can even create a neck that doesn't exist. Neck length and jawline must be carefully considered in the face picture.

Shoulders: What do shoulders have to do with face shape? A lot, I think. If you have big, wide heavy shoulders and a short muscular neck, a short, short geometric haircut may make you look very silly. And if you have a mane of hair in layers that cascades for days you'll look just as silly. Your shoulders determine your body's proportion, and your hair must be in proportion to your body. The jaw, neck, and shoulder connection is particularly important. Small people should not have too much hair bunched around narrow shoulders and a tiny face. Wider shoulders set off more hair.

Now let's take a look at some examples and combinations, to see how it all works together.

Long face, oval jawline: The emphasis should be on fullness on all sides. Bangs are almost a must—they can cut a too-long face almost in half, which is essential here. Fullness on all sides will make the long face appear to be an oval. But remember, no fullness on top, because this will only serve to lengthen the face.

Long face, pointed chin: You need fullness in the middle, but keep it rounded at the jaw. Avoid any styles with points. Harsh geometric cuts are all wrong—go for soft and full.

Long face, square jaw: Brush the hair away from your face on the sides, at the square part of the jawline.

Oval face, oval jaw: You can wear almost any style. Look to the other features on your face for direction—nose, forehead, neck, and so on.

Oval face, pointed jawline: You will need soft, full hair at the jaw and neck. Do not pull your hair back or away from your face. You can wear any style on top, but make sure the sides come in along the jawline and stay soft along the neck. Short severe cuts and geometric cuts are not for you.

Oval face, square jawline: Brush the hair away from your face at the temples and keep it soft and flattering. A wide bang will square your face more, so try to avoid this. You are wearing a soft bang or a partial bang that sweeps up. Your hair should frame your face and neck to keep the jawline from overpowering your face.

Round face, oval jaw: Because of its fullness, you need to lengthen the look of your face, so add some height on top with either short hair or short layers that can fluff up. You can wear almost any style, as long as you don't make your face look any rounder.

Round face, pointed jawline: The chin cuts your round face and makes it look what some people call heart-shaped. Balance this with soft full hair that frames the jawline and neck without making your face look too round. You will need height on top to accomplish this. Long hair with some height is one possibility.

Round face, square jawline: Your face is very wide, and you need both height and length. Bangs should be lifted up, and the hair at the temples should not go out too far. You can wear length and width at the jaw and neck.

HAIR TYPE; HAIR KIND

So many times I talk with women, and they say to me that they want a hairstyle like such-and-such a movie star or someone whose photograph they saw in a magazine, and then they show me the picture and I think it's a joke. The person in the picture has an entirely different type of hair from the woman who is showing it to me. Never in a million years could I make this woman happy. Oh, sure, I could probably duplicate the look in the salon. But she wouldn't be able to do it at home, and it wouldn't be practical for her life-style. Women with curly hair always want straight hair. Women with straight hair always want curly hair. It's like the old saying about the grass's always being greener—very few women are satisfied with what God gave them.

But I can tell you now, the best way to be happy with yourself is to accept what you do and don't have and learn to enjoy it. That's what makes each person special. If your hair type calls for a certain style, don't fight it. Have the style cut for your face picture and accept your hair type with grace.

I break hair type into two categories: hair type and hair kind. I know that sounds silly to you, but here's what I am thinking:

Hair type is curly, frizzy, or straight.

Hair kind is dry, oily, or a combination.

Hair kind has very little to do with the styling of your hair and can usually be corrected with treatment.

Hair type can be altered some of the time (a permanent can make straight hair curly; curly or frizzy hair can be straightened or relaxed chemically), but if you want to keep your life as simple as possible, you'll change your hair type to match your life-style. A permanent may change your life!

Besides hair type and hair kind, let's throw in *hair body*. There are three types here also: thick, fine, and normal. Hair body is usually not related to the condition of the hair and may or may not be related to hair type, though most wavy, curly hair is thick. But you cannot generalize too much here, and the ability of your hair to last in a style is related to its hair-body measurement.

Now let's figure out your hair type, so you can find the variables that pertain to you. Please put down this book and take a shower. If you don't want to take a shower, you can go to the bathroom (or kitchen) sink and completely wet your hair. I think a shower will be easier, darling. Leave the book in front of the bathroom mirror, and when you come out of the shower, pick up where you were.

Welcome back. Now, please towel-dry your hair just a little bit, to get the extra moisture out. Run a big comb through your hair, to get it smooth and without tangles. If you normally put a part in it, do that now. Now I want you to wait. Every ten minutes or so, go to the mirror and check your hair. As it dries, you will see how much curl it does or does not have. Within twenty minutes you will know if it is straight, wavy-curly, or frizzy.

Now comb out a strand of hair to the side of your head. Let it fall from the comb's teeth back to your head. How fast does it fall? The faster it falls, the straighter it is. And the finer. This is your hair-body measurement.

Hair Body

Thick Hair

Thick hair has to be cut just so, or it can stick out on the sides and make your head look twice as big as it is, or, worse, make it look like it's a funny shape. So the more layers you have, the better, especially underneath and at the bottom. A blunt cut is not right for you unless you want to look like Cleopatra. And you should never have your hair thinned with the razor. A razor cut would be very bad, because hair grows back in too many directions. If you like the one-layer look, you can have your hair layered very slightly in a really subtle way, and it will look all one length but will behave better.

Mostly, the layers in the haircut should be adjusted to your face shape. You should avoid a permanent or just get a mild one or a body wave, so that the chemicals are concentrated on the roots, because that's the part that's flat. A body wave at the roots can give your hair a little lift. Thick hair is usually heavy, and the weight can pull the curl out, so you may need this extra help at the roots.

Thick hair should be maintained carefully and cut every four to six weeks. Cut is extremely important, and you must take pains not to let the cut grow out of control.

Fine Hair

Fine hair is the absolute contrary of thick hair. It can be blunt cut, but it shouldn't be one length, because layers will make it look thicker. If it's done right, a permanent can be a good way to add some volume. I'd say eighty percent of the women with this kind of hair need a body wave or a permanent to give the illusion of fullness. Fine hair should be cut with a scissors, never with a razor. Coloring will make fine hair thicker, and yes, color and permanent can be combined if they are done professionally.

I recommend bangs for fine hair. Then you don't have to worry about your hair having enough body to stand up or stay teased. A good haircut is important because the style will not stay if you rely on rollers or hair spray.

Normal Hair

When you have normal hair body, you can have whatever you want. If there is not enough body, you can get a permanent. Whatever your face shape needs you can do easily.

Frizzy Hair

Frizzy hair is tightly curled. Black people have frizzy hair, and so do a lot of white people. Frizzy hair has its own special texture—the curl is so tight that it doesn't even

15

wave. Frizzy hair is kinky all the way to the roots and is curled so tightly that it shrinks when you touch it. You can never even accurately determine how long the hair is, because it's curled so tightly. So for frizzy hair, the haircut is extremely important but very difficult. Short hair can look good when it is done well; even extremely short hair is good if you have the right face shape and bone structure. You can blow-dry frizzy hair and use a round brush to help pull the frizz out. You can also use a curling iron. I know this sounds ridiculous to you, but it's true. Heat takes the frizz out, and the curling iron gives you wonderful control and a nice soft curl. If you have frizzy hair you should never try to straighten it, because it is never going to look right, darling, and it will always be expensive and time-consuming, and it's bad for your scalp to use harsh chemicals.

If you have frizzy hair, learn to live with it and love it. But don't ever use electric rollers. They will give you too much volume. Heat helps, but not too much. The curling iron is your best bet—use the heat to straighten the roots and to softly curl the ends.

If you really want to, you might have a treatment called "relaxing," but please don't do this more than two or three times a year. You'll burn your scalp and make the condition of your hair very bad. If, after two months, you think you need another treatment, go buy yourself a new dress instead. Wait another two months before you do anything. Even when the advertisements tell you that the chemicals are not too strong, do not believe them. Even "soft" soft-hair relaxants are too strong to use more than three times a year.

Conditioning is going to be very important, whether you use a relaxant or not. You must condition frizzy hair on a regular basis. You should use a creme rinse after you shampoo, and then once or twice a month take time out for a heavy conditioning. Spend thirty to sixty minutes with conditioner on your hair, wrapped in tin foil. Sit under the hair dryer and read magazines or do your nails.

If you have frizzy hair and you want to wear it long, you must be very careful that it is layered and kept in shape. Otherwise you will look like a bush!

When you have frizzy hair you should experiment with style and be adventuresome. Accept your hair as part of yourself and wear it long, short, with bangs, or in any new fashion styles you want. Don't be afraid! And try hair accessories for extra fun. You can look very exotic without much trouble.

Wavy-Curly Hair

If you have wavy-curly hair, you are very lucky—you have the hair that everyone wants. Lots of women with this kind of hair tell me they have hated it all their lives. I say, darling, be happy now. Everyone else is getting a permanent. For the last five years everyone has wanted hair that has wave or curl. You are very lucky. And if you want straight hair, you can have it. The blow-dryer can make your hair perfectly straight. Electric rollers can give you more curl and body for a special occasion or particular styles. You can have anything and everything, and your hair can do whatever is necessary to suit your face.

Straight Hair

Straight hair is missing the body and bounce that your dream hair will have. But you can have these things with a permanent, so don't despair. There are many different types of permanents, and one of them will work for your kind of straight hair, depending on its body and your face shape and your life-style needs. Some straight hair is thick and some is thin. Thin hair must be treated very delicately so it doesn't break off. If you have straight hair and you want a permanent, you definitely should not do it at home.

With straight hair the emphasis has to be on the roots, so that your hair just doesn't hang there. If you don't want a permanent, sponge rollers are very good for straight hair. So are tissue papers, See page 197. You don't have to have a permanent to get curl. Try bobby pins. Try juice cans. Try wrapping. See page 35. Straight hair can take on any personality you want it to have. Enjoy!

Hair Length

Hair length as a variable is more a question of life-style than anything else, because almost every facial shape can wear almost any hair length if it is cut right. However, there is one really big myth about hair length that I am going to dispose of right here and now. The myth is that most people think short hair is easier to handle or fix or make look good quickly just because it is short. So many women tell me that they want short hair because they are going on a trip, or having a baby (if they are having a baby, I can usually tell without their saying anything), or they have no time. Sometimes they even say they want short short hair, like a boy's, because they think this is the easiest way to care for. Well, I hope this won't upset you too much, but this information is wrong.

To me, the easiest, quickest, best hair length for any face shape and any life-style is medium. Medium-length hair with a light permanent is wonderful—you can step out of the shower, the hair dries naturally, and *voilà*—it goes into place and you look gorgeous. What could be more easy than that?

Short hair can be very difficult to work with. Listen to me for a minute and then think about it.

You must have the right face shape for short hair. And the shorter the hair, the more perfect your face must be.

Short hair needs more upkeep, because it must be cut every three–four weeks. If you are busy, how do you have time to go to the beauty shop so often? If you aren't rich, can you afford this?

Short hair looks bad when it's messy, so it's less versatile, especially if you are in a hurry. Long or medium hair can always be pinned up, tied back, or fluffed up into a soft, sexy tangle of curls. End of speech on short hair.

I put most hair lengths into three different categories, to keep things simple.

Short hair is above the chin.

Medium hair is above the shoulders.

Long hair is at least shoulder-length.

Obviously, there's very, very short hair and there's very long hair . . . and maybe there's very medium hair, but I don't think so. You have to be very young, or looking for a really dramatic image, to have extremely long hair, and many times there is not too much you can do with it. (Remember Cher's long hair? It was her trademark, but she wore a lot of wigs to get versatility.) While I don't think that age and hair matter too much, and there are a lot of silly rules about these things, you should be young to wear very long hair.

On the other hand, many women think that if you are over thirty-five or forty, you can't wear long hair. This is wrong, darling. We'll talk more about age in a minute, but basically you can wear whatever hairstyle is becoming to you, and age has nothing—nothing whatsoever—to do with it. Often for women over forty, I recommend long hair, especially for women who have the life-style that gives them enough time to do anything with their hair (Life-style Blue). You can do more things with long hair than with any other kind of hair, so it is the most versatile in terms of the styles and looks a woman can master. But you have to have the time for this.

Generally, though, I recommend medium-length hair. If you are a Life-style Red or Green, medium-length hair is probably just right for you. The best thing about medium hair, after all, is that it's very medium.

AGE

I hear so many myths about age and hair that I don't know where to start to straighten all this out. I've already told you to forget the idea that you can't wear long hair if you are over thirty-five or forty. You just shouldn't wear long, long hair, like a hippie. So I've already thrown out myth number one.

Myth number two is that you start losing your hair when you are old. You can lose hair at any time in your life, for any number of reasons. Aging doesn't necessarily mean a loss of hair. If you find that your hair is thinning, consult your doctor. It could very well be your diet. I'm sure it's not your age.

Myth number three is that hair changes texture when you have your change of life. I haven't found this to be true. Sometimes hair texture changes as a woman grows older; other times it does not. Hormonal changes do affect hair growth for some people, and they may affect hair texture. But this is an individual thing. You can grow old without any change in your hair, believe me. (Ronald Reagan says he doesn't even color his hair, so age may not even affect hair color!)

Hair can change, and there are many reasons for the changes. But you cannot say that when you become forty or fifty or sixty your hair will change because of the aging process. I have seen thick hair turn thin, dry hair become oily, straight hair grow curly. But these changes are not due to the passing of a certain number of years. If your hair is changing, consult, first your hairdresser, then your doctor. It could be your diet, it could be medication, or it could even be pregnancy.

As people get older I find they accept a lot of things without questioning them and turn them into stereotypes. You think that if you are a grandmother you have to look like a grandmother. This is wrong. You are only as old as you look and feel. If you're sixty but you look forty, then the world sees you as forty. Every hairstyle is possible for you when it fits your face. Generally people will say that short hair is better as you age, but I think that's true only half of the time. Short hair lifts the face, but you'd be amazed at how young you can look with long hair. It all depends on your face, your life-style, your attitude. If you are older and opt for longer hair, I suggest the hair be styled to lift away from the sides of the face. As you age it is more flattering to have your features show, even if you have wrinkles. They give you character. You earned them, so you should flaunt them. If you try to hide them with hair, you will look ridiculous. When you try to hide something, you only accentuate it. You want instead to frame the face by pushing the hair back and away, with a lift at the temples.

You should never have full heavy bangs unless they are part of your trademark look and you haven't changed your hairstyle in fifty years. Moderate bangs are okay, but as you get older, the softer the style, the better it is for you, darling. Avoid the severe unless it's your hallmark.

HEALTH AND NUTRITION

Have you heard the expression that you are what you eat? Well, so is your hair. Just like your nails, your hair is a product of your good health or your ill health. Whatever you put into your mouth affects your nails and your hair. And while you can purify your body in a matter of hours or days, of whatever bad things you put into it, your hair has a six-month memory. So if you eat junk foods, darling, or do not treat your body well, your hair will be telling the world about it for at least six months.

If you're on a crash diet or a fad diet or if you are fasting, the results will be showing on your head. If you eat well-balanced meals, if you exercise, if you are healthy and don't take drugs (I don't mean just Hollywood drugs; I mean Valium or even lots of aspirin or birth-control pills or even medication prescribed by your doctor for a particular ailment), you will have strong, healthy hair that will reflect the state of your whole body.

Nutrition

Nutrition is a matter of what and how you feed your body. While you may eat one nutritional meal, it takes three to make the day—you're not supposed to be skipping meals, remember? The way you eat, what you eat, what time you eat it, and the water you drink—as well as the soft drinks and the booze and whatever else you might drink—all affect your body and your hair.

Shine and luster come from within. No hairdresser can make unhealthy hair beautiful. Just as your own inner glow comes from within you and depends on your mental health, the shine and true condition of your hair depend on your physical health—and what you eat.

Water is an important part of nutrition. I suggest that everyone drink a lot of water during the day. I drink Perrier. But the water you drink doesn't have to be bottled; you should just drink a lot of it. If you travel a lot, you know that changes in water can affect the condition of your skin and your hair.

If you ever have a question about your nutrition and the ability of your hair to reflect your total body plan, go to a doctor who does hair analysis. The doctor will take a snip of your hair (don't be alarmed if he asks for your pubic hair; it's more pure) and send it to a lab. The lab will come back with a detailed report of the things that your body is lacking or getting too much of. This report can even diagnose disease and see the potential for illness. And most labs only charge about $30 for this test.

I can't give you a big lecture on nutrition, because I am not a doctor, but I know, from the hair I look at all day, that improper nutrition and an imbalanced diet will do things to hair that even I cannot fix. If you have damaged hair that conditioners cannot cure, talk to your hairstylist. Ask him if you need to see a nutritionist or a medical doctor. But don't decide on a cure yourself. Too many vitamins can damage your hair just as much as too few. You can go overboard on a health kick and hurt your health.

Health

Health as a state of body is often related to nutrition, although not necessarily. You can eat perfectly balanced meals and still get a cold; it happens all the time. And believe me, excessive amounts of cold pills or aspirin can show up in your hair. If you get the flu and take prescription drugs or if you have a more long-term illness, you can expect to see a change in your hair.

And any drug that affects your hormones will definitely affect the way your hair grows—and doesn't. Many women who take the Pill tell me that globs and clumps of their hair come out each time they wash their hair. This is very common for pill-takers and is not really a serious problem (you won't end up bald), it just clearly indicates the power of medication to change your hair.

WEATHER

Very few people ever take weather into consideration when they are picking a hairstyle or deciding what to look like that day. They know that weather affects their mood, and they think of seasonal changes in terms of haircuts. Every spring my clients want me to braid flowers in their hair, every summer they want short hairstyles, and every Christmas they want their hair long and full. So climate, mood, and hairstyle are all very much interrelated.

The climate where you live should be something you think about when you pick your hairstyle. A hairstyle is a living, breathing thing. What it looks like in a magazine or the salon is meaningless. But if you pick one that is right for your life-style and your face shape and does not go with the weather, you may be cursing your hometown whenever the weather changes.

Let's assume that you have found the style that is right for you and that four times a year—for each of the seasons—you like to update that style a little bit. That means you may cut it a little shorter at the beginning of summer and you may leave it a little longer for the fall and holiday season. Now go through this checklist, season by season, and ask yourself these questions about your hairstyle and its compatibility with the weather where you live.

- Is winter so cold that you wear a hat or a scarf to keep warm?
- Is winter so cold that your hair will not dry in half an hour?
- Is winter dry and windy? Does your hair need extra conditioning?
- Is summer hot and humid? Do you get the frizzies?
- Are you out in the sun a lot, and is your hair covered?
- Do you play sports activities in the sun? In the wind? In the cold?
- Does your hair color change in the sun? Does its condition change?
- Does the altitude affect the ability of your hair to hold curl or a set?
- When it rains, does your hair frizz? Go limp?

If you live in a cold climate, where winter lasts several months, you will be wearing a warm hat every time you go outdoors. Some women wear a silk scarf tied tightly under their chin, but lately I've been seeing fur hats, Lawrence of Arabia turbans with a scarf attached, and little-boy yarn caps that pull down almost to the nose. (Few women wear a felt hat in this kind of weather, because it can blow away and it doesn't cover the ears or keep them very warm.) Even though you're warm, your hairstyle is usually ruined by these hats. So you need to think of snow and cold and wind and ice and pick a soft, probably curly, hairstyle that can stand getting crushed by the weight of a hat or scarf, if you want to look instantly perfect when you pull off your *chapeau*.

If you have hair that frizzes in the rain or in humid weather, relax. There is only one thing you can do: enjoy your hair. Let it do whatever it wants, and try liking it instead of hating it. You can stand in the bathroom for an hour and get your hair perfectly straight with a blow-dryer and then step outside, and, within five minutes, find your hard work is ruined. You want to cry. You want to hide. You want to stay home that day and pray to the weather god. None of this is necessary. You need to learn to love what you've got and let it be free. Short of covering curly hair with a thick gel and slicking it back against the head, nothing will keep your hair in a man-made style. So collect hats and accessories that will help you look fashionable and chic. And forget about taming the frizzies. Then you can be free to be you and to smile. Be pleased with yourself; feel gorgeous, and you will be radiant. No one will care whether your hair is straight or frizzy.

If your hair has been colored, you must also take the weather into consideration, for two reasons: the sun can damage your colored hair, and sun damage can cause you to have to color your hair (which can be damaging if your hair is not in good shape). Let's make that a little simpler.

First of all, say you color your hair all the time. In the fall and winter months your hair is an even and consistent medium brown. You may do it yourself or have it done in a salon; it doesn't matter. It is always even and simple, and no one knows that you have more gray hairs than you would like to admit. Then it gets to be spring—say May—and even though you have not been sunbathing, you see that your hair is a little more red than usual. It's a nice color, so although it's different than usual, you don't worry about it, because it's nice and it's natural and it's not brassy or anything vulgar. But as the summer progresses, your hair turns redder and redder. While you still use the same process on your hair, month after month, something has gone wrong. Sunlight is causing oxidation, and so the color changes. And if you sunbathe, that is even worse. Both condition and color deteriorate very quickly.

And if you are a blonde, the process is even more ugly. Sun can turn color-treated blonde hair any shade from orange to green. This does not mean that if you want to color your hair, you cannot live in a sunny climate—but you must make sure your hair is covered and particularly take care of it when you sunbathe, sail, play tennis, or are exposed to sunlight for longer than an hour. (That even means driving in a convertible, darling.)

Generally, people like long hair for extra warmth in the winter and short hair for cool, casual breeziness in the summer. I find that longer hair is easier for summer, because you can pull it back and stick it under a hat to protect it. Shorter hair, medium length, maybe, is better in winter, because it dries more easily and quickly (you shouldn't go to bed with a wet head) and can be revitalized more easily when you take off all the layers of hats and scarves and things that keep you warm. So think about it next time a big seasonal change is coming.

WIGS

Some people think of wigs as a variable of their hairstyles and fashion looks. I don't. Unless you are a movie star, I'd like to steer you away from wigs. I don't think they are a good variable. To me, almost always, a wig looks like a wig. And you should have a hairstyle that is so easy, you don't need to improve your look with something that is not you.

There is only one reason that I am in favor of a wig, and this is medical. I hope that nothing like this ever happens to you, but it does happen to some people, so let's talk about it for just a minute. Some medications, especially the chemotherapy used in cancer treatment, may make your hair fall out. You may feel perfectly all right without hair (I have seen some women who look stunning!), but probably you will be feeling sick and uncomfortable already and won't want people to stare at you; you'll want to look as normal as possible. Then you should get a wig. In this case it should be as good a wig as you can afford. Even though your hair will grow back in a few months, the better the quality of the wig you buy, the more real it will look on you and the less people will ever notice your predicament. If you get a cheap wig that does not fit properly, you will be even more uncomfortable, worrying if people can tell you are wearing a wig.

Remember, it's a lot easier to secure a wig to your own hair than it is to a thinning or bald pate, so make sure your wig won't be sliding around.

When it's time to pick the wig, wait as long as you can. Getting the wig before you need it may make you feel a little more secure psychologically, but the wig you try on with a full head of hair may fit very differently when your hair begins to fall out. When that happens, find someone who knows a lot about wigs and a lot about hair (such as your hairdresser), and who will be able to give you good advice at what may be an emotional moment.

Be sure that you get a hair color and style that is much like what you've been wearing, so that no one will notice the difference. This is not the time to suddenly go platinum blond. A small change in style is recommended, because then, if people notice that you look a little different, you can always say it's the new hairstyle. (That's why you should always change your hair a little after you've had plastic surgery, too—people will notice the change and attribute the new look to your hairdresser, not your surgeon.)

MOOD

Mood is a very intangible thing, but it often has something to do with your change of hairstyle and haircut. Mood may even influence your score on the life-style test. (You should take the test twice, by the way, a few days apart.) Mood and hairstyle are kind of like Catch-22: your mood can influence your style, and your style can influence your mood.

How you feel about yourself is definitely reflected in how you look. You may be the most beautiful woman in the world, but if you are unhappy or do not have self-confidence, you will not be very attractive. Even your beauty will be empty. But if you are plain or homely and you feel great about yourself, you can be radiant and gorgeous and wildly attractive. That's because a lot of beauty comes from inside yourself, and whatever your own self-image, it is reflected in your hairstyle.

If you think you are chic and elegant and you wear blue jeans and a t-shirt but you are impeccably made up and you stand straight and carry yourself like a princess and your hair is groomed marvelously, then your mood will come out of your head and through your body and will touch the world around you, and everyone you meet will know you are a person with style.

If you act unsure of yourself, you end up looking that way.

And if you are unhappy with yourself, you will never be pleased with what you see in the mirror—no matter how perfect you may be.

While hair is a very real thing, because it is part of beauty it has also psychological depth. Your hairstyle can affect your mood, and vice versa. And this has nothing to do with optical illusion.

Many times customers come to me and say that they want something special for that night—they have a new boyfriend or they are going to a party where they want to be noticed or they want to make a good impression or they have a job interview—and for a moment or an evening or a small while they want to be somebody else. Then they want a certain look.

And this is one of the things I'm best at. Because these women almost always want to look more glamorous and sexy than they dare to in their normal lives, I can help them. I can feel the fantasy wish coming from inside them, and I know that, while they may be shy about it, they want to come out of themselves a little bit.

I have seen women come into the salon looking like athletes and leave looking like sex queens. And once I fix their hair differently, they begin to change themselves in subtle ways. A dramatic hair change allows you to play a role, and while you may not want to change your personality for life, it is something that is fun for an evening or to suit a special dress or occasion.

By the same token, if you come to me in a bad mood and you ask for something terribly dramatic to get you into a better mood, chances are, it will not work. I never suggest that anyone go to the hairdresser in a bad mood. If you do, don't make a big change. You may be sorry later, and you will probably blame it on the hairdresser.

It seems that every time a women breaks up with her lover, she cuts her hair or changes its color. She should probably buy a new dress instead. You can make a change on the spur of the moment, but you have to be in a good enough mood to shrug your shoulders and say, "It will grow," if you are not pleased with the results.

YOUR PERSONAL WORKSHEET

Susie Coehlo was one of my first clients. She brought Farrah to me and sent me so many of her actress and model friends, so I have been doing her hair for a really long time. Susie is a model who is also an actress. She has long hair that is naturally curly, and she is very exotic-looking and glamorous. She likes a natural look, but she can be anything, with hair and makeup changes; this is one of the things that makes her such a terrific model. She also has a very good knowledge of her face and its features and of how to coordinate her features with her hairstyle and her life-style. So I asked her to fill out a personal worksheet, to give you an idea of how to do it. After you read hers, it's your turn, darling. You be as honest as Susie. And don't worry if you don't look like her. You're not supposed to be comparing yourself to the women in this book. You're supposed to learn how to take their secrets and make them work for you—when applicable!

PERSONAL WORKSHEET

name ___Susie Coehlo___

My face shape is: round   (oval)   long

My best feature is my: _eyes_

My worst feature is my: _tits!_

My eyes are:

color ___dark brown___

size ___small___

shape ___almond___

special features ___My eyes are my best asset, so I like them to look as big as possible.___

I wear glasses: yes   (no)

If yes: infrequently   part of the time   all of the time

I would like my eyes to appear (bigger, smaller, more dramatic, etc.) _Big and round and innocent; sexy_

Choose as many as fit:

My cheekbones: don't show   (are pronounced)   _I have big hollows_

(are high)   are flat   are wide   (are narrow)

My mouth: large   (small)   thin lips   thick lips   pouty lips

(bow lips)

My ears: stick out   (lie flat)   big   (small)   (pierced)

not pierced

My nose:

size ___small___

shape ___slightly upturned___

special features ___it doesn't have any, I'm lucky___

_122,772_

25

My nose is the focal point of my face: yes   (no)

My forehead is: high   low   (average)

I have a widow's peak: yes   (no)

I wear bangs: yes   no   (some of the time)

My jawline is: wide   narrow   (square)   (oval)   *Slightly squared chin*

Draw your jawline on top of the face shape that best suits you:

round   oval   long

Makes sort of a heart

My neck in proportion to my shoulders:

The two are equally balanced: (yes)   no

My shoulders are small; my neck is longer: (yes)   no   *My shoulders are wide, but my neck is longer*

My shoulders are wide; my neck is short: yes   no

My hair type is: (curly)   (frizzy)   straight

If combination, what combination: _____

My hair kind is: dry   oily   (normal)   combination

My hair body is: thick   (fine)   average

My hair length is: ___ *long*

My hair condition is: ___ *excellent*

Medications and treatments that may affect the growth and condition of my hair:
I don't drink or smoke or take the Pill
_____
_____

My eating habits are: irregular   (excellent)   average   *I drink a lot of water and watch what I eat.*

I am out in the elements a lot: yes   (no)

My hair is covered when I am outdoors: yes   (no)

My hair color is: (natural)   one-process   two-process   *henna sometimes*

I have a permanent: yes   (no)

I have both perm and coloring: yes   (no)

PERSONAL WORKSHEET

name _____

My face shape is: round   oval   long

My best feature is my:

My worst feature is my:

My eyes are:

color _____

size _____

shape _____

special features _____

_____

I wear glasses: yes   no

If yes: infrequently   part of the time   all of the time

I would like my eyes to appear (bigger, smaller, more dramatic, etc.): _____

_____

_____

Choose as many as fit:

My cheekbones: don't show   are pronounced

are high   are flat   are wide   are narrow

My mouth: large   small   thin lips   thick lips   pouty lips

bow lips

My ears: stick out   lie flat   big   small   pierced

not pierced

My nose:

size _____

shape _____

special features _____

My nose is the focal point of my face: yes   no

My forehead is: high   low   average

I have a widow's peak: yes   no

I wear bangs: yes   no   some of the time

My jawline is: wide   narrow   square   oval

Draw your jawline on top of the face shape that best suits you:

round   oval   long

My neck in proportion to my shoulders:

The two are equally balanced: yes   no

My shoulders are small; my neck is longer: yes   no

My shoulders are wide; my neck is short: yes   no

My hair type is: curly   frizzy   straight

If combination, what combination _____

My hair kind is: dry   oily   normal   combination

My hair body is: thick   fine   average

My hair length is: _____

My hair condition is: _____

Medications and treatments that may affect the growth and condition of my hair:

_____

_____

_____

_____

My eating habits are: irregular   excellent   average

I am out in the elements a lot: yes   no

My hair is covered when I am outdoors: yes   no

My hair color is: natural   one-process   two-process

I have a permanent: yes   no

I have both perm and coloring: yes   no

YOUR PERSONAL PRIORITY LIST

We all have priorities in life, and sorting them out seems to make the most important things happen. Some people are able to have a hairstyle that fits their lifestyle, their faces, and every other need in their life. Other people (most people) are not so lucky. For them, a priority list is a must.

Go through all the variables I discussed in Part Two and then list, in the order of your individual priorities, the things that are most important to you. When you show this list to your hairstylist, he will have a better idea of the things he must accomplish for you.

For example, if you live in Houston, Texas, and you have hair that frizzes, the most important priority for you may be weather. First of all you will be looking for a hairstyle that will not frizz—or is so frizzy, the weather can't disturb it. Weather may even be more important to you than your face shape. For someone else, a face shape will be a top priority, and weather will be way down on the list—or not on the list at all. Try to rank all the subjects in the variables section—even your age—so your hairstylist can help you the most.

Each person's hairstyle must be crafted from the elements that are most important to her, so gather all the information and then organize it. *Then use it.*

PERSONAL PRIORITY LIST

Rank

_____ Face Shape

_____ Hair Type

_____ Hair Body

_____ Hair Length

_____ Age

_____ Health

_____ Weather

Part Three:

THE LIFE-STYLES

Life-style Red

PROFILE

You don't have to be an Aries to be living the Life of Red. You don't even have to be in the red financially, or seeing red when you're angry. You might not dress red—you don't need to, darling: you live a bold, fast, and furious life, and you deserve every free minute you get. But I know you well, and you rarely have a free minute.

A lot of my celebrity ladies are Life-style Red, because they live such hectic lives. Whoever thinks all a movie star has to do is lie back on silk pillows and eat bonbons has been reading the wrong fan magazines. Most movie stars lead the same kind of life as mothers of small children! Every day they are running around doing something different—frequently going to many places in the same day, always wanting to look good but often not having time for a touch-up or a fluff-up before the next stop. And you thought it was all chauffeurs and glamour. The typical celebrity client who tests Red is usually up at 6:00 A.M. to be on a set all day. Or she has a breakfast meeting with an agent, a morning meeting at a studio, a lunch date with a producer, an afternoon filled with fittings and makeup, and then may have evening plans in which being seen is very important! And because everyone expects a star to look good all the time, somewhere in between she has to fit in exercise class, dance lessons, or some vigorous activity that will keep the pounds off the thighs. This will inevitably cause her to perspire—and she'll need to wash her hair and redo her makeup.

For the real-life woman who is not a celebrity, the day is fraught with just as many activities. The Red woman is usually a housewife or a woman who works for herself. She does not go to an office and sit at a desk, generally speaking. She probably uses her home as her office and dashes in and out to meetings or to do errands and so many different types of activities that it's impossible to say where she will be going next or what is the right look for any one activity. I also put athletes into the Life-style Red, because they have to make such drastic changes in their performing or practicing life and their life off the court or out of the pool or off the track.

And invariably all these women have to wash their hair more than once a day. They may, in fact, be washing their hair two or three times a day and bathing just as often. This is not good for you. If you must, wash your hair two times a day, but once is better, and *never* wash more than twice. There are some tricks I will teach you to help you look fresh and keep grease- and sweat-free without a total washup. Too much washing is bad for your skin and your hair, and damaged goods do not look their best.

The Life-style Red woman is usually up bright and early in the morning, without the aid of an alarm clock. She may not be a morning person by nature, but her obligations (such as her children!) have her trained to early rising, so it's second nature to her now. And because she's up and running, she never sets aside quite enough morning time for her own beauty rituals—she grabs moments to herself whenever she can, or she's filled with good intentions. Some days she has more time than others; some days she looks better than others; but there's no consistency to her look, especially in the mornings, and she wakes up wishing she were a natural beauty who looked instantly and carelessly gorgeous.

For the Life-style Red woman, the best kind of hairstyle compliments her face shape and is still wash-and-wear. She needs a cut that requires no attention, and she may want to have a permanent—but not necessarily. She can wear her hair any length, depending on the other variables in her life, and hair accessories are her best friend.

With wash-and-wear hair, darling, believe me, after one month you can get very bored looking at the same thing all the time. And versatility is what makes a woman feel good. So if you play tennis, take advantage of all the fashion accessories, sweatbands, visors, caps, and anything else that will make you feel good about your appearance and change the way your hair looks, while leaving it flattering. Combs, combs, combs are also important—don't use your old rubber band darling; pin up your hair with two or three combs. Who cares if it falls partway down in half an hour?—that's a charming way to look. Combs will also be helpful for evenings, especially since you probably won't have time to fix your hair with hot rollers or a curling iron. Also scarves, turbans, headbands, silk flowers, and hats of all kinds are accessories that the Life-style Red woman should be collecting.

One of the worst problems the Red woman has is her tendency to look too *sportif* with her hairstyle or to think that she has to have a short, short haircut. This is all wrong. The Red woman does have choices, and if short hair is wrong for her face, then it is no good for her life-style. We've already talked about the myth that short hair is best for quick-and-easy life-styles. So don't forget it now.

Because the Life-style Red woman is so busy, she often forgets to get her hair cut on a regular basis. She may also have roots showing on her hair before she gets it colored, and never has time for a professional manicure. She needs to be very organized about her beauty appointments—highlighting or streaking, which doesn't leave roots, is probably better for her. Nothing looks worse than roots!

If you are a Life-style Red because you are a sports buff or an athlete (or even a woman with a heavy athletic-activity schedule), make sure that you take care of your hair during your sporting activity. If you are out in the sun, take the trouble to wear a hat. If you swim, use a bathing cap. If you don't wear one, take plenty of time rinsing your hair when you get out of the pool, because the chlorine in the water will do terrible things to your hair. If your hair is colored or permed (or both), be very careful. I wouldn't want to see you walking around with green hair. It's not very chic this season, believe me.

Many Life-style Red women are so health-oriented that they don't like to put chemicals on their hair and are very cautious about what they eat. They know that, as I said before, you are what you eat, and good-looking hair is based on good nutrition. There are other Life-style Red women who are so busy running around that they don't take time to eat sensibly, and too many candy bars or too much junk food can show in the hair.

But then, why should I bother to give a speech? Life-style Red women don't take the time to listen. They are like the wind, whipping around in all directions, dressed in bright colors or jazzy neutrals, women of fashion who won't be dictated to but are persistently on top of trends or gravitate to the snazzy and slightly unconventional. Yet they're still practical about the way they dress—they may want cashmere sweaters and lace ruffles, but they know those things don't suit their life-style, so they try to stay sensible when choosing their wardrobe.

If the Red woman is a mother of young children, she's also into being practical. She passes up real silk for the fake stuff, knowing that washability is essential at this time in her life. She carries an inexpensive handbag so that if it gets ruined, she won't be heartbroken. But she's usually got a few nicer bags for special occasions or evenings. When I see her, she is almost always carrying a big canvas tote or a shopping bag filled with the necessities of her life. She may even have a diaper bag on one shoulder!

Because the Life-style Red woman can do so many things, she's usually pretty good at fixing her own hair—she just doesn't take the time to do it. She's got at least one set of electric rollers, and she regularly buys whatever new appliances she thinks will make her life easier. (But in the end, she rarely uses any of them.) In fact, she's a big fan of natural drying, and would like to avoid taking the time out to use a blow-dryer. She rarely has the time—or patience—to stand for half an hour or an hour to brush and style her hair to be the way it would in the salon. This woman is the perfect example of someone who looks good in the beauty shop but cannot manage her own look herself. She needs to be very careful when picking a style and must be honest about the amount of time she's going to devote to her beauty routine, so she can look her best—and she can look divine, I promise—with the investment of only a little time and effort. Even though Life-style Reds are so busy, they are the type of people who tackle extra jobs and are always there to help out friends; they are always willing to do something extra. In fact, they spend a lot of their time thinking of other people, and if they have some extra money, they will probably use it to buy something for someone else rather than themselves. Reds are by nature very giving people, and it's this very fact that can undo them, beauty-wise—they are so busy doing for other people that they take time away from their hair and makeup. It's not that they don't want to look good, but their hair is a low priority compared to the demands of the children or the needs of other people.

Life-style Reds are, therefore, very people-oriented. They rarely sit home and read a book on a slow night. It's not that they choose to party all night—invariably they are early risers and go to bed early—but they do like the company of others. Reds like to go to football games, to be involved in family activities, and to socialize with all their friends.

HOW TO SHAMPOO YOUR HAIR

Basically, all people should shampoo their hair the same way; after all, there is a right way to do it. It's not something that varies much with life-style. But I have found that there are a few tricks that do depend on the style of living, so I want to pass them on to you, and maybe you can use them.

For the Red woman who knows that the next day is going to be so busy that she will not have time to wash her hair—or who realizes that her schedule can be made better if she eliminates washing her hair—the trick is to wash the hair the night before and merely wet it or spray it with a water-spritzer bottle (the kind that people spray on plants to give them moisture) until the hair takes shape. If you have oily hair, this is not a very good technique, because your hair may be too greasy early in the afternoon for you to look respectable, and you don't want to wash your hair twice a day if you can help it. But for most hair types, this shortcut is worth trying as often as two or three times a week. Just don't go to bed with a wet head in the winter, darling!

I tell everybody to shampoo in the shower, because I think this is easier, unless you have a built-in professional sink in your home and your own shampoo boy. Usually shampooing in the sink is awkward and gives you a sore back and neck. And it doesn't get your hair as clean as it should be. Even if you are a bath person and you have a European shower-hose, I still think the shower is the best place for a good hair wash. And for a Red woman, who seldom has the time for a luxurious bath and is in and out of the shower all the time, it's perfect.

First rinse your hair in lots of water—not so hot that you burn your scalp or make your head secrete its oils too fast (which can make your hair get dirty more quickly), but it needn't be tepid either. (Some people, especially Reds, like cool or cold rinses.)

Pick a soft shampoo. I won't name brands, but I do suggest that you pick two or three shampoos that you like and rotate them, either daily or by the bottle. Soft means mild, to me, because when you are washing your hair every day, you want a mild shampoo. Do not use too much shampoo, and only shampoo once. I do not think you need a double sudsing unless you have spent three weeks on a camel in the desert with your hair uncovered. (Then you need professional help for your head as well as your hair!)

Use a lot of water when you shampoo, but remember that suds are not the important thing. Massage the shampoo into the scalp with your fingertips (not your nails) in a rotating, circular motion. Be sure to work over the entire scalp and your hairline.

Rinse thoroughly. And I mean thoroughly: for two or three minutes. You don't have to have a cold rinse for the last thirty seconds, but many people like it. It does help to produce a better sheen, and some experts say the cold stuns the oil glands into closing down production, so hair becomes dirty less quickly.

Many Life-style Reds have to wash their hair twice a day, or they think they do—once when they wake up in the morning and once after an athletic event or before an evening event. I do not recommend shampooing twice a day, and I prefer if you use the spritzer trick we talked about for later in the day. Or you can wash the hair at night before bedtime, and then wash it without shampoo (just give it a good rinse) after the sporting event.

Whatever you do, don't wash three times in one day! (And don't tell me you don't see how that's possible. If you're a Red, you know it's simple: early in the morning, after sports, and before the evening's entertainment . . .)

Because you are washing your hair so often, you have to be very careful about conditioning.

CONDITIONING

According to the amount of dryness in your hair, you should have deep or heavy conditioning once to twice a week. This is when you use a cream product or oil-treatment conditioner and then wrap your hair in aluminum foil or a towel and leave it for twenty-thirty minutes. Life-style Reds always groan at this part, but really it's very simple—you do it while you are watching television with the family, or making the children's lunches for tomorrow, or sorting the laundry. After your hair is wrapped in aluminum foil, cover it with plastic or a shower cap and then put on a scarf or turban. That way, your boyfriend or your husband or your children will not make fun of you. You can rinse out the conditioner after half an hour and then towel-dry your hair and save shampooing until the next morning. See? Anyone, no matter how busy, can do this once or twice a week.

If your hair is permed, colored, washed twice a day, and treated to a dose of sunshine or chlorine, you are going to need deep conditioning more than once a week if you want to have healthy, good-looking hair. One good thing about Reds is that they don't have too much time for blow-dryers and electric rollers or curling irons, so they don't damage their hair that way.

You can use creme rinse when you shampoo, but you don't have to worry about using too much of it, like Life-style Greens do. Their hair must last all day and have more body and staying power than yours. But remember that the creme rinse goes mostly on the ends (not the roots) and if you will be sweating or out in the sun, go light on creme rinse, because you don't want to muck up your hair so that it needs to be washed any sooner than you can help it!

HOW TO DRY YOUR HAIR

Since the Life-style Red woman will seldom stand still long enough to style her hair fully with a blow-dryer, she needs several tips for wash-and-wear hair drying. Her cut (with any luck) is so in tune with her face-shape and hairstyle variables that when the weather conditions are right, she can run her fingers through her hair and walk away from the bathroom without a care in the world. Mother Nature and fresh air will do the rest.

Another good way to dry the hair, if you have a little time to sit down (you can do something else while you're sitting there), is with an infrared-heat lamp. The beauty salons have expensive gooseneck ones that the stylist positions around you almost like kleig lights, so you get a good dry. But you can buy an infrared light bulb and put it in a metal art-director's lamp that clips on and is adjustable so you can get the right angle for wherever you choose to sit. If you've got about twenty minutes (unless your hair is really long), you can get your hair almost dry with this treatment, then fluff it with your fingers and let it dry the rest of the way by itself.

If you do happen to have long hair, one of the better ways of drying it may be the wraparound method. Wrapping is a very American technique and is popular with people who don't have a lot of time to straighten their hair or even to set it with rollers, but who don't want to let their hair dry naturally, for fear that it will kink and curl too much and be very wild and have no shape. When you hair-wrap, you are giving your hair just enough curl, because the curl comes from the curves of your head.

Hair wrapping is for long hair only! If your hair is not long enough to go around your head at least once, don't even try it.

Your hair must be wet in order to wrap it properly. So:

1. Wash or spritz your hair till it's completely wet.
2. Apply setting lotion if you want a little extra oomph and body. Setting lotion will also help straighten naturally curly hair.
3. Carefully comb through your hair.
4. Make a part on the left or right crown.
5. Moving in the direction of the part, wrap the hair against the head as tightly as possible. Clip it with long, skinny metal clips to hold it flat. Do not use little clips, as they will leave marks.
6. Pull and stretch your hair as you wrap it around, making sure it lies smoothly. Bumps and squiggles will show up when the hair dries.
7. Wrap it completely around your head as many times as possible.
8. Let it dry. Unpin it. Comb it out. (Do not sleep on wrapped hair.)

The wraparound method is particularly good if you wash your hair at night, wrap it around your head while it's damp, and let it dry before you go to sleep. Don't go to sleep with a sopping-wet wrapped head, because whatever way you sleep will make an indentation on top of your hair! And for the wrap to be effective, make sure it's done smoothly. Don't get impatient on this job, or you will have the frizzies. But to tell you the truth, I don't think I've ever met a Life-style Red who wrapped her hair. These women don't have the time or patience for it.

Life-style Reds should always have a blow-dryer on hand, although, if they're lucky, they won't have to use it. In the wintertime, of course, when you cannot rush about with damp hair, a blow-dryer is a necessity. The best way to dry your hair is to fluff it up with your fingers and rotate the blow-dryer through it. Be sure to dry your hair from underneath; this will assure you of not having wet roots (which is why you don't want to go into winter air with wet hair—the ends dry quickly enough by themselves; the roots take longer) and will also help your hair appear to have more volume. In fact, you can bend over and dry your hair sort of upside down, and this will give you the most fullness. Shake your hair as you go, and you will get soft, sexy, full hair that is messy, but controlled enough to be styled, and it will take less than ten minutes from your busy schedule.

PERMANENTS

In some cases, I recommend a permanent for a Life-style Red because it helps in the wash-and-wear department. But it is not a necessity and really depends on the style and condition of the hair. Reds often abuse their hair, so if your hair is already colored and you wash it twice a day, I'm not sure that I would suggest a permanent for you. It all depends. A good cut is more important than a permanent in this case.

COLORING

Coloring is applicable to any life-style. For Reds, the benefits of color are that it does give hair more body, which will probably make it easier to fix, and more wash and wear. Because Reds are so busy, they have to worry about ugly roots growing out, so I recommend highlighting, hair painting, or one of the natural types of coloring that fades a little with each shampoo, so it doesn't really leave any roots.

TO SPRAY OR NOT TO SPRAY

If you are a Life-style Red, darling, I don't even want to see a can of hair stray in your home. Hair spray can be very damaging to hair, and I don't like anyone to use it. And it is a really big mistake for Reds. If you are a true Red, you are very, very active, and hair spray will just gum up your hair. Your hair should have bounce and life and freedom, so if you spray it, you will look all wrong. Please, I beg you, forget about hair spray.

SUPPLIES

Daily
soft shampoo (several varieties, to alternate)

Often
creme rinse
deep conditioner
aluminum foil
blow-dryer

Occasionally
combs
barettes
veils
silk flowers
hats
visors
headbands

YOUR MORNING SCHEDULE

- 6:30–7:00 A.M.: Wakeup
- Other activities (tending to children, phone calls, exercise, sports,): 30–90 minutes
- Shower and wash hair: 10 minutes
- Fluff and finger-dry hair with ligh blow-drying: 10 minutes
- Makeup: 5–7 minutes
- Dress for the day: 2–3 minutes

- Total beauty routine: 30 minutes
- Total morning routine: 60–90 minutes

Maud Adams

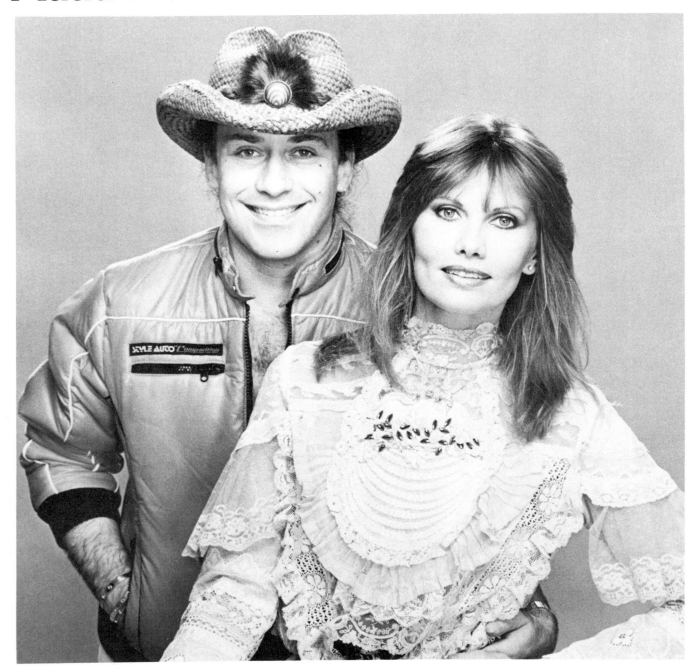

I moved to L.A. about three years ago and I realized I was going to need a good hairdresser for maintenance. I asked a lot of people whose hair I admired and who had similar life-styles where to go, and time after time the same name came up: Jose. So I went to him.

The marvelous thing about working with Jose is that he's an excellent technician, but more importantly, he understands his clients. He doesn't try to impose his will on them; he lets his clients decide what they want. It's a joint venture. You tell him what you need, and he has an intuitive understanding of how to give you what you want in the way that's best for your face and your hair. And then he seems to be able to sense when you're ready for a change. More than anything, he has a wonderful way of being able to translate what you want to what is right for you.

I wash my hair every day; I condition it a lot. And that, along with a good haircut, is all I need.

JOSE EBER'S LIFE-STYLE QUIZ   *Maud Adams*

1. **When I wake up in the morning:**
   A. I look at the alarm clock and panic. I'm already late.
   (B.) Who needs an alarm clock? I'm up with the birds, or the kids, and ready to go.
   C. I roll over and go back to sleep for another half hour because last night really was a bit too much.

2. **My regular morning routine:**
   A. Takes no more than half an hour because I'm so busy.
   (B.) Is postponed until later in the day, because I'm out the door for tennis or carpool.
   C. Depends on what I'm doing during the day and what's cooking for the upcoming evening.

3. **When I look in the mirror each morning I:**
   A. Wish I had time to do something about what I see.
   (B.) Splash cold water on my face and check the condition of my skin.
   C. Study each line, blemish, and soft spot mercilessly, until I'm satisfied I know exactly how to best care for what I've seen.

4. **First thing in the morning, my hair:**
   A. Needs a wash and blow-dry.
   (B.) Kind of falls into place, because my haircut is easy to care for.
   C. Is almost perfect, because I just had it done yesterday.

5. **My hair:**
   A. Gets cut whenever I'm in the mood or can't do a thing with it.
   (B.) Needs to be cut every four–six weeks; otherwise it's unmanageable. *Sometimes it's longer, but generally true.* It's long to allow me to manage a variety of hairstyles depending on my needs so I just make sure the ends are trimmed frequently. *that*

6. **My hair color:** *It's a combination of B and C; I alternate,*
   A. Is something I like experimenting with myself. *But when I have it colored I go to a professional*
   (B.) Yuck! Ruin my hair with chemicals?
   C. Is done at the beauty shop every six weeks.

7. **The colors I wear most frequently are:**
   A. Neutrals that mix well in the business world: navy, burgundy, cream, and things that are "safe."
   (B.) Bright colors, I love 'em.
   C. Whatever the fashion mavens say is "in." As long as it's always flattering to my skin tones. *Sometimes it's A, depending on my mood*

8. **For a purse, I usually carry:**
   (A.) One good all-purpose bag that goes with all my clothes.
   B. Something fun and inexpensive that holds all the junk I carry around.
   C. Whatever matches my clothes.

9. **The hair appliances I rely on include:**
   A. A round brush and blow-dryer.
   (B.) I have all kinds of stuff, but I never use it.
   C. Electric rollers, hairpins, combs, clips, curling iron, crimper, dryers, and brushes.

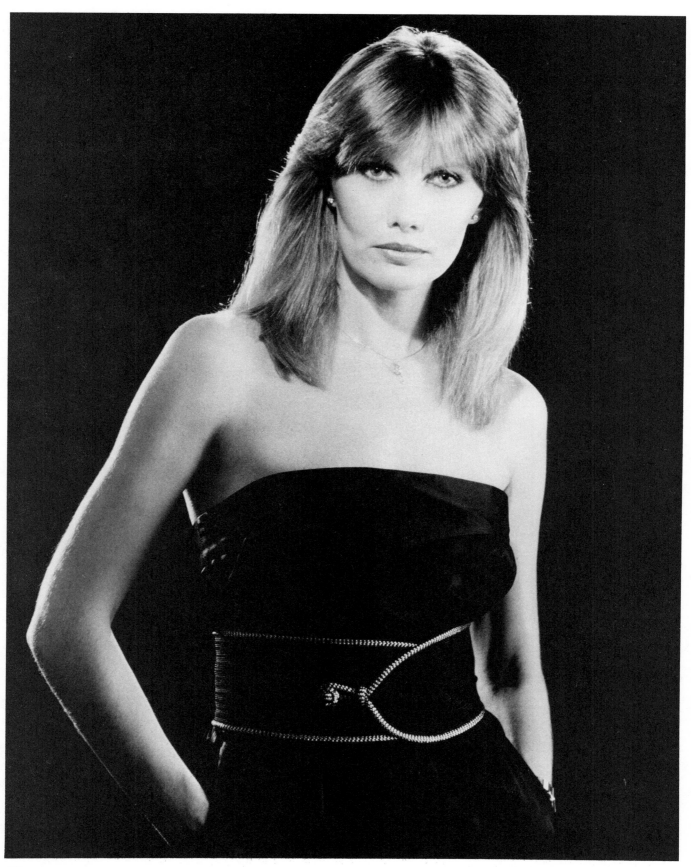

10. **For breakfast, I:**
    A. Grab something on the way to work or eat at my desk
    B. Have cold cereal and fruit.
    C. Eat a light meal if I'm dieting or a little more if I'm having a late lunch.

11. **When I bathe, I:**
    A. Take a shower first thing in the morning. *B and C, really*
    B. Take a shower several times a day, after tennis or swimming.
    C. Take a leisurely bath.

12. **I have help in my home:**
    A. Never.
    B. Once or twice a week.
    C. Full time.

13. **I put myself together:**
    A. To please myself. *all three, actually.*
    B. To suit my life-style.
    C. To please my man.

14. **I work:**
    A. Nine to five at a regular job.
    B. You think taking care of the kids isn't full-time work?
    C. Flexible hours or not at all.

15. **My fingernails:**
    A. Are manicured by me.
    B. Are kept short and neat for simplicity.
    C. I have done weekly.

16. **When it comes to athletics:**
    A. Weekends are the only time I have for recreational sports.
    B. I'd only be more active if I were training for the Olympics.
    C. I don't sweat.

17. **If I have a little extra money to splurge with, I:**
    A. Buy something I need. *B and C*
    B. Get something for the kids.
    C. Buy something wonderful I've been dying to have.

18. **My idea of the perfect vacation would be to:**
    A. Travel to the major cities of Europe.
    B. Go hiking and backpacking.
    C. Escape to a spa. *A and B, but not together!*

19. **My bedtime is:**
    A. After the 11:00 P.M. news.
    B. Early, after an exhausting day.
    C. Whenever the party's over.

20. **If I could sum up my beauty routine simply, I would say it's:**
    A. Sensible.
    B. Practical.
    C. Time-consuming.

Stockard Channing

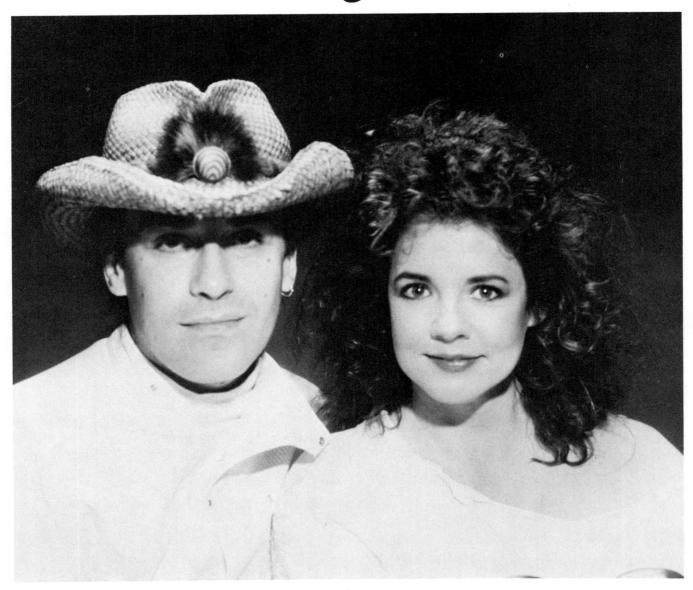

I was terrified to go to Jose. Basically, I've always hated most hairdressers, and going to them is awful. But when Jose gave me a cut, I wished I had come to him years before.

I met Jose because two of my friends went to him, so I decided to give it a try. I'm used to doing my own hair and makeup, because in the theater you do that, so you get stubborn about it. A lot of hairdressers want to do to you whatever they want, and there's no give and take between you. Even if you tell them what you want or expect, they ignore you and do their own thing. Jose isn't like that. I have problem hair, but Jose can do my hair, and he respects what I have to say about it.

It's crazy hair. It's baby-fine and it needs a lot of work, whether I do it or someone else does it. If I'm going out, after I wash my hair I dry it and then use the curling iron. If I'm just staying home, I squeeze my hair in place with my fingers and let it dry naturally. I like to have width around my eyes and not have it too high on the top. I have big cheeks, and I need my hair to be cut in a shape that follows my head.

I'm careful about conditioning it, and I have the morning routine worked out around the conditioner: I get in the shower, wash my hair, and put on the conditioner. Then I get out of the shower and make the coffee. Then I go back into the shower to rinse off the conditioner, and when I get out, the coffee is already brewed.

JOSE EBER'S LIFE-STYLE QUIZ

Stockard Channing

1. **When I wake up in the morning:**
   A. I look at the alarm clock and panic. I'm already late.
   B. Who needs an alarm clock? I'm up with the birds, or the kids, and ready to go.
   C. I roll over and go back to sleep for another half hour because last night really was a lends too much.

   all three, well, it depends, plays and movies call for different schedules.

2. **My regular morning routine:**
   A. Takes no more than half an hour because I'm so busy.
   B. Is postponed until later in the day because I'm out the door for tennis or carpool.
   C. Depends on what I'm doing during the day and what's cooking for the coming evening.

   I spend about twenty minutes in the bathroom, then ten minutes, for fifteen minutes and do some stretching exercises.

3. **When I look in the mirror each morning I:**
   A. Wish I had time to do something about what I see.
   B. Splash cold water on my face and check the condition of my skin.
   C. Study each line, blemish, and soft spot mercilessly, until I'm satisfied I know exactly how to best care for what I've seen.

   D. I don't look in the mirror at all unless I'm making up my face.

4. **First thing in the morning, my hair:**
   A. Needs a wash and blow-dry.
   B. Kind of falls into place because my haircut is easy to care for.
   C. Is almost perfect, because I just had it done yesterday.

   I wash my hair every morning in the shower.

5. **My hair:**
   A. Gets cut whenever I'm in the mood or can do a thinning with it.
   B. Needs to be cut every four–six weeks; otherwise it's unmanageable.
   C. Is long to allow me to manage a variety of hairstyles depending on my needs so I just make sure the ends are trimmed frequently.

   I do have it trimmed every six weeks. But I do cut it myself.

6. **My hair color:**
   A. Is something I've experimented with myself.
   B. I touch up my hair with chemicals?
   C. Is done at the beauty shop every six weeks.

   But it varies from season to season because my hair is exposed so the color changes with the seasons and it needs a lot of care.

7. **The colors I wear most frequently are:**
   A. Neutrals that mix well in the business world: navy, burgundy, brown, things that are "safe."
   B. Bright colors, I love.
   C. Whatever the fashion mavens say as long as it's also flattering to my skin tones.

   Colors depend on the climate. In New York I wear blacks, tones, peach and pale because the light is different. I have to wear bright, harsh, new wave colors or prints.

8. **For a purse, I usually carry:**
   A. One good all-purpose bag that goes with all my clothes.
   B. Something fun and inexpensive that holds all the junk I carry around.
   C. Whatever matches my clothes.

   D. It's sort of A but it really depends on what I'm doing normally I carry one large bag with a lot of papers and books.

9. **The hair appliances I rely on include:**
   A. A round brush and blow-dryer.
   B. I have all kinds of stuff, but I never use it.
   C. Electric rollers, hairpins, combs, clips, curling iron, crimper, dryers, and brushes.

   curling iron, period. I travel a lot.

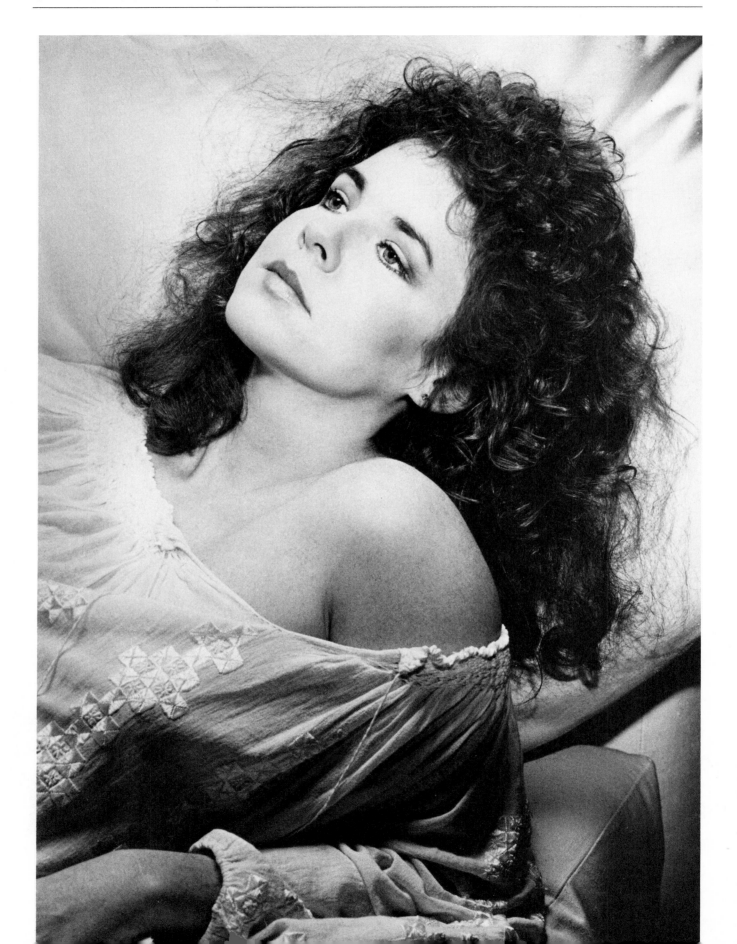

10. For breakfast, I:
    A. Grab something on the way to work or eat at my desk.
    B. Have cold cereal and fruit.
    C. Eat a light meal if I'm dieting or a little more if I'm having a late lunch.

    Fresh squeezed orange juice and coffee.

11. When I bathe, I:
    (A.) Take a shower first thing in the morning.
    B. Take a shower several times a day, often after tennis or swimming.
    C. Take a leisurely bath.

    Maybe a bath in the evening, but that's training. Rare.

12. I have help in my home:
    A. Never.
    B. Once or twice a week.
    C. On weekends.

    Depends on where I'm living, but I don't have full time help.

13. I put myself together:
    (A.) To please myself.
    B. To suit my life-style.
    C. To please my man.

    All three, actually.

14. I work:
    A. Nine to five at a regular job.
    B. You think taking care of the kids isn't full-time work?
    C. Flexible hours or not at all.

15. My fingernails:
    A. Are manicured by me.
    B. Are kept short and neat for simplicity.
    C. I have done weekly.

    D. I have them done irregularly. I have the worst nails in the world and I try not to look at my hands!

16. When it comes to athletics:
    A. Weekends are the only time I have for recreational sports.
    (B.) I'd only be more active if I were training for the Olympics.
    C. I don't sweat.

17. If I have a little extra money to splurge with, I:
    A. Buy something I need.
    B. Get something for the kids.
    C. Buy something wonderful I've been dying to have.

    D. I never shop. I guess I might take a trip if I had some extra money, unless someone I know needed it.

18. My idea of the perfect vacation would be to:
    (A.) Travel to the major cities of Europe.
    B. Go hiking and backpacking.
    C. Go spend a month in France.

    Europe, but not necessarily the major cities. I wouldn't mind a trip to Provence in France.

19. My bedtime is:
    A. After the 11:00 P.M. news.
    B. Early after an exhausting day.
    C. Whenever the party's over.

    whenever I want. God, I'm self indulgent. Of course I'm working, it's another story.

20. If I could sum up my beauty routine simply, I would say it's:
    A. Sensible.
    (B.) Practical.
    C. Time-consuming.

    It's not C. I guess it's A or B. B, practical.

Jose says:
Stockard likes to keep her face looking slim, so we surround her with hair. Her hair is very fine, but she has lots of it, and it's naturally curly. So the top is cut shorter, to get the right volume to balance out the rest, and her face is framed perfectly by a lot of natural softness.

Cathy Lee Crosby

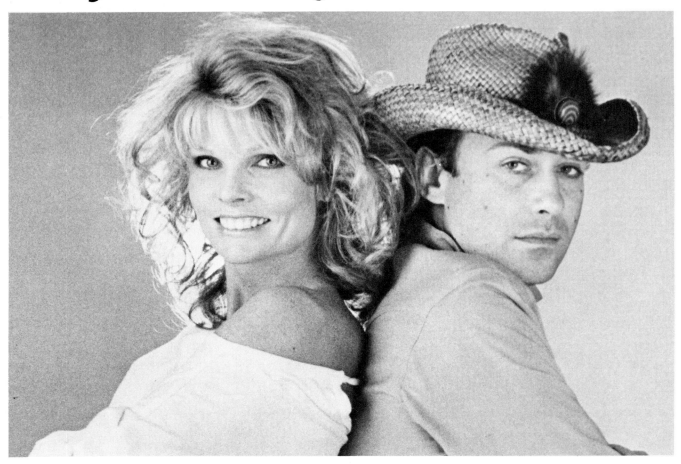

I met Jose when I had to do a commercial and I was absolutely panicked. I had no hair and I asked several people to recommend a hairstylist to me. Both Cher and Farrah suggested Jose. Two days before I was to go in front of the camera, I went to Jose and said, "Help me!"

Immediately I knew he could, and that he was right for me. I felt totally at ease and very beautiful and very sexy when I left. Two days later, when we shot, Jose made my short hair bushy and full and wonderful, and I felt good about it.

The first day I met him, his opening remark to me was, "Darling, you have no hair, but we're going to fake it until it grows." And that's what we did.

I fiddle around with my hair, but it's really Jose's decision. And Araxy has helped a lot. She's given me healthy hair. When I first came in, Jose took me by the hand and walked me upstairs to where Araxy works. She reworked my color. She brought back life to my hair. She has a recipe for a conditioner that's been in her family for centuries. It's amazing. My hair was broken and poorly cut and damaged and colored improperly. It was a mess. But now I'm back in shape, thanks to Jose and Araxy.

Now I go to the shop and just hang out. If Jose is busy, I do my hair myself—I snip at my bangs. I watch at the shop a lot and then I imitate. I've noticed that to get the hair bushy and full, Jose turns the rollers up instead of down, so I do that now too.

There's another side to Jose that no one else will mention and he won't tell you about, so I'd better. I did a special called, "Get High on Yourself," and Jose gave his time and did everyone's hair free, because it was a show about drug abuse. And one Christmas, on a Monday, when the shop was closed, Jose opened it for Cher and a bunch of kids she brought in from MacLaren Hall, and he gave a free haircut and perm to every kid. He does a lot of charity work like that, which no one knows about, and I think he should get some credit for it. He has a big heart and a good sense of humor, and those are two things that are really important to me.

JOSE EBER'S LIFE-STYLE QUIZ   *Cathy Lee Crosby*

1. When I wake up in the morning:
   A. I look at the alarm clock and panic. I'm already late.
   (B.) Who needs an alarm clock? I'm up with the birds, or the kids, and ready to go.
   C. I roll over and go back to sleep for another half hour because last night really was a bit too much.

2. My regular morning routine:
   A. Takes no more than half an hour because I'm so busy.
   B. Is postponed until later in the day, because I'm out the door for tennis or carpools.
   C. Depends on what I'm doing during the day and what's cooking for the upcoming evening.

[handwritten: Doesn't exist — nothing is my routine! Life is my routine or I get bored!]

3. When I look in the mirror each morning I:
   A. Wish I had time to do something about what I see.
   (B.) Splash cold water on my face and check the condition of my skin.
   C. Study each line, blemish, and soft spot mercilessly until I'm satisfied I know exactly how to best care for what I've seen.

[handwritten: I throw water on and moisturize and go.]

4. First thing in the morning, my hair:
   A. Needs a wash and blow-dry.
   (B.) Kind of falls into place, because my haircut is easy to care for.
   C. Is almost perfect, because I just had it done yesterday.

[handwritten: It falls into place, but I still wash it every morning, because I love clean hair.]

5. My hair:
   A. Gets cut whenever I'm in the mood or can't do a thing with it.
   B. Needs to be cut every four–six weeks; otherwise it's unmanageable.
   C. Is long to allow me to manage a variety of hairstyles depending on my needs so I just make sure the ends are trimmed frequently.

[handwritten: I cut it as little as possible because I'm growing it out.]

6. My hair color:
   A. Is something I've experimented with myself.
   B. Yuck! Ruin my hair with chemicals?
   (C.) Is done at the beauty shop every six weeks.

[handwritten: It's done regularly but not streaked — I just have the front dark; blond and basically the rest is my natural color.]

7. The colors I wear most frequently are:
   A. Neutrals that mix well in the business world: navy, burgundy, cream, and things that are "safe."
   (B.) Bright colors, I love 'em.
   C. Whatever the fashion mavens say is in, as long as it's also flattering to my skin tones.

[handwritten: I love pastels and but I love black and vibrant colors too.]

8. For a purse, I usually carry:
   A. One good, all-purpose bag that goes with all my clothes.
   B. Something fun and inexpensive that holds all the junk I lug around.
   C. Whatever matches my clothes.

[handwritten: I like a lot of different kinds of funky bags — not necessarily cheap or expensive or meant to match my clothes.]

9. The hair appliances I rely on include:
   (A.) A round brush and blow-dryer.
   B. I have some kinds of stuff but I never use.
   C. Electric rollers, hairpins, combs, clips, curling iron, crimper, dryers, and brushes.

[handwritten: and sometimes hot rollers.]

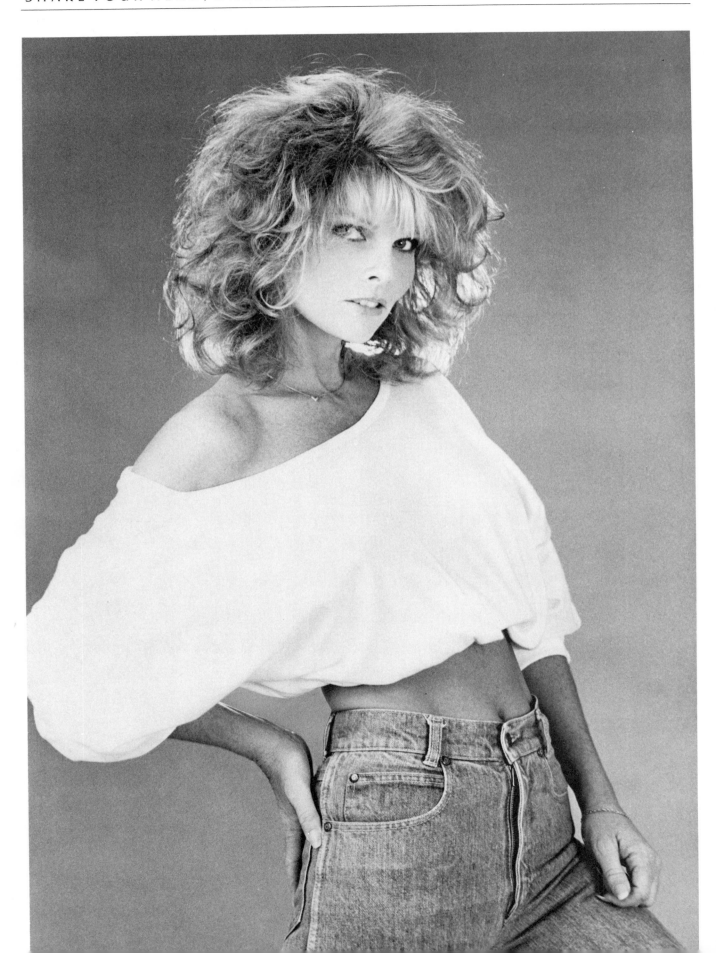

10. For breakfast, I:
   A. Grab something on the way to work or eat at my desk
   (B.) Have cold cereal and fruit.
   C. *something warm half a grapefruit, a piece more if I'm dieting, for a warm more having toast off lunch.*

11. When I bathe, I:
   A. Take a shower first thing in the morning.
   (B.) Take a shower several times a day, after tennis or swimming.
   C. Take a leisurely bath.
   I like to do all three.

12. I have help in my home:
   A. Never.
   (B.) Once or twice a week.
   C. Full time.

13. I put myself together:
   (A.) To please myself.
   B. To suit my life-style.
   C. To please anyone.
   Basically A but really A and B. Never C.

14. I work:
   A. Nine to five at a regular job.
   B. You think taking care of the kids isn't full-time work?
   C. Flexible hours or not at all.

15. My fingernails:
   A. Are manicured by me.

   B. Are kept short and neat for simplicity.
   (C.) I have done *I have them done regularly* them *is that every two weeks not* done. *But every two weeks not every week.*

16. When it comes to athletics:
   A. Weekends are the only time I have for recreational sports.
   (B.) I'd only be more active if I were training for the Olympics.
   C. I don't sweat.

17. If I have a little extra money to splurge with, I:
   A. Buy something I need.
   (B.) Get something for the kids.
   C. Buy something wonderful I've been dying to have.
   It's B and C

18. My idea of the perfect vacation would to:
   (A.) Travel to the major cities of Europe.
   B. Camping and backpacking.
   C. Escape to a great spa.
   It's A with someone I love on a great romantic holiday. But I'm going to an island. It has to be romance, or it's no vacation. I'm a dyed-in-the-wool romantic.

19. My bedtime is:
   A. After the 11:00 P.M. news.
   B. Early, after an exhausting day.
   C. Whenever the party's over.
   All three.

20. If I could sum up my beauty routine simply, I would say it's:
   A. Sensible.
   B. Practical.
   C. Time-consuming.
   None of those. My beauty look is such a small part of my life, it's a joy.

. . . .

Jose says:
Cathy Lee has extremely fine, baby-fine, hair. She has it streaked, so she cannot have a permanent. To get the fullness and the wildness that she likes in her hairstyle, we cut the hair several different lengths. She likes a hairstyle that doesn't look done, and we get this look by cutting her hair in very irregular lengths. We tease it very lightly and use hot rollers some of the time. We set the rollers going in all different directions, so the hair is wild and full. Then it is combed to frame the face and show off the cheekbones. There are some bits of hair that fall on the forehead, but we don't really call these bangs; they just give the look some extra snap.

Jamie Lee Curtis

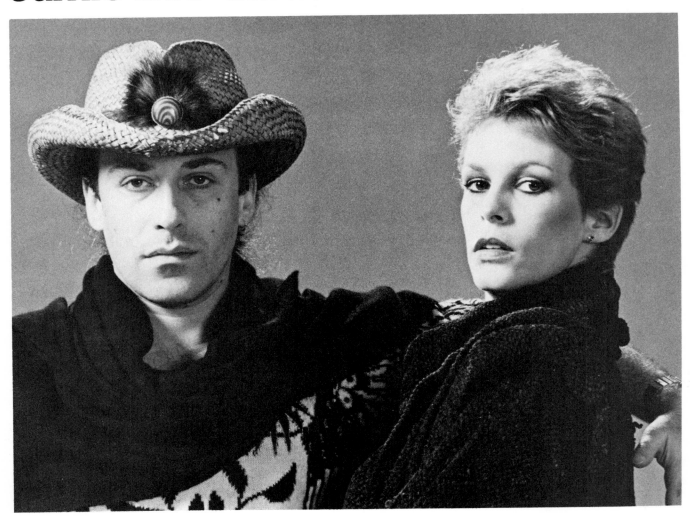

Let me tell you about my hair. The hair on my head is very fine. I've had to have it colored for a lot of different roles, and it was dyed platinum blond for a television film, "The Dorothy Stratton Story." My naturally brown hair had to be bleached, not once, not twice, but three times—count them, three times. Then, after the film, I decided to have my hair dyed brown again so it could grow out to my natural hair color. I was in New York, right after this film, and it was a really vulnerable time in my life. I went to a hair dresser for the coloring. He suggested that I get a perm. Knowing I shouldn't, I did, and it turned out like straggly pubic hair. Honest.

Within two days, the crown of my head was balding. My hair literally broke off about one inch from the scalp. Every time I touched my head, more hair broke off. I went to lunch with my manager, and she personally took me by the hand and led me to Jose. I went from the point of hair suicide—I felt like I had cancer—to this. I just looked at Jose and said, "I'm yours." He cut my hair to one inch long, and I never felt better in my life. I got a lot of compliments, and now it's the easiest part of my anatomy to deal with—and it used to be the most difficult. And I've got a look with style that I never had before. I would recommend this kind of haircut to anyone who can wear it. It suits my life-style, and my hair went from being a pain in the ass to something that's really fun.

JOSE EBER'S LIFE-STYLE QUIZ

Jamie Lee Curtis

1. When I wake up in the morning:

A. I look at the alarm clock and panic. I'm already late.

B. Who needs an alarm clock? I'm up with the birds, or the kids, and ready to go.

C. I roll over and go back to sleep for another half hour because last night really was a bit too much.

D. I sleep like a rock but I'm never late because I use five alarm clocks, all over the room.

2. My regular morning routine:

A. Takes no more than half an hour because I'm so busy.

B. Is postponed until later in the day, because I'm out the door for tennis or carpool.

(C.) Depends on what I'm doing during the day and what's cooking for the upcoming evening.

3. When I look in the mirror each morning I:

A. Wish I had time to do something about what I see.

B. Splash cold water on my face and check the condition of my skin.

C. Study each line, blemish, and soft spot mercilessly, until I'm satisfied I know exactly how to best care for what I've seen.

D. I laugh.

4. First thing in the morning, my hair:

A. Needs a wash and blow-dry.

(B.) Kind of falls into place, because my haircut is easy to care for.

C. Is almost perfect now because I just had it done yesterday.

Especially now because of Jose.

5. My hair:

A. Gets cut whenever I'm in the mood or can't do a thing with it.

(B.) Needs to be cut every four–six weeks; otherwise it's unmanageable.

C. Is long to show off. It needs a variety of hairstyles depending on how I feel.

Since I have manager short hair, it needs constant cutting and attention to keep it in shape and looking nice.

6. My hair color:

A. Is something I've experimented with myself.

B. Yuck! Ruin my hair with chemicals?

C. Is done at the beauty shop every six weeks.

D. I don't do anything, except when I'm working.

7. The colors I wear most frequently are:

(A.) Neutrals that mix well in the business world: navy, burgundy, cream, and things that are "safe."

B. Bright colors, I love 'em.

C. Whatever the fashion mavens say is "in," as long as it's also flattering to my skin tones.

8. For a purse, I usually carry:

A. One good all-purpose bag that goes with all my clothes.

B. Something fun and inexpensive that holds all the junk I carry around.

C. Whatever matches my clothes.

D. Abercrombie and Fitch fishing bag

9. The hair appliances I rely on include:

(A.) A round brush and blow-dryer.

B. I have all kinds of stuff, but I never use it.

C. Electric rollers, hairpins, combs, clips, curling iron, crimper, dryers, and brushes.

51

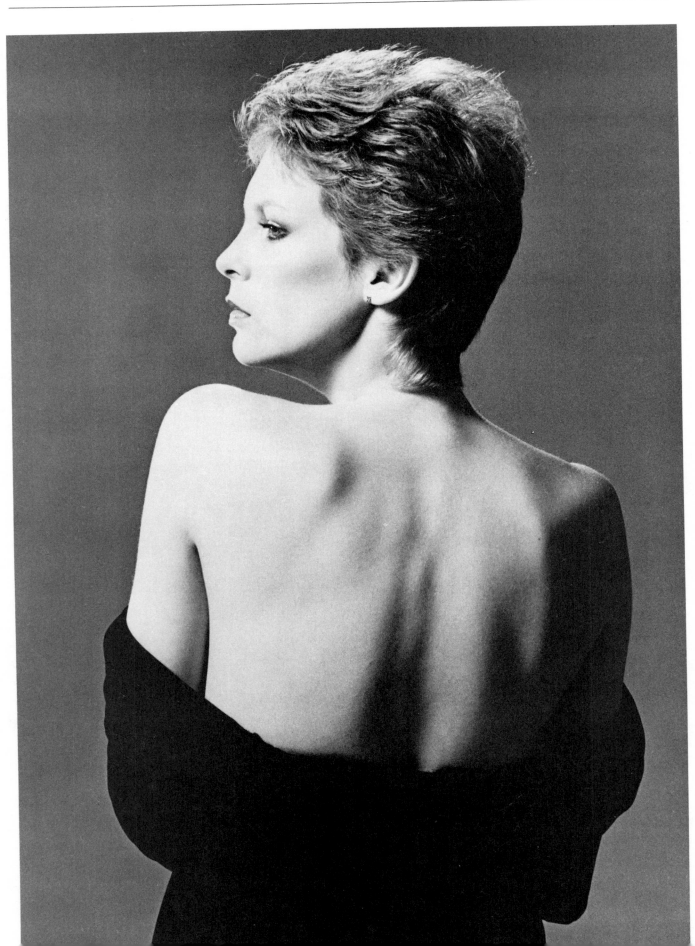

10. For breakfast, I:
A. Grab something on the way to work or eat at my desk
(B.) Have cold cereal and fruit.
C. Eat a light meal...

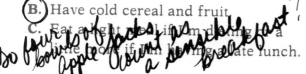

Do four bowls of Apple Jacks count as a sensible breakfast?

11. When I bathe, I:
(A.) Take a shower first thing in the morning.
B. Take a shower several times a day, after tennis or swimming.
C. Take a leisurely bath.

12. I have help in my home:
A. Never.
(B.) Once or twice a week.
C. Full time.

Once a week: Thursdays.

13. I put myself together:
(A.) To please myself.
B. To suit my life-style.
C. To please my man.

A, B, and C.

14. I work:
A. Nine to five at a regular job.
B. You think taking care of the kids isn't full-time work?
C. Flexible hours or not at all.

15. My fingernails:
A. Are manicured by me.

B. Are kept short and neat for simplicity.
C. I have done weekly.

But no matter what I do to them they're always dirty.

16. When it comes to athletics:
A. Weekends are the only time I have for recreational sports.
(B.) I'd only be more active if I were training for the Olympics.
C. I can't sweat.

I don't have time for my face, except for my body. If I do aerobics but that's just my body for two and a half hours every day.

17. If I have a little extra money to splurge with, I:
A. Buy something I need.
(B.) Get something for the kids.
C. Buy something wonderful I've been dying to have.

18. My idea of the perfect vacation would be to:
(A.) Travel to the major cities of Europe.
B. Go hiking and backpacking.
C. Escape to a spa.

19. My bedtime is:
(A.) After the 11:00 P.M. news.
B. Early, after an exhausting day.
C. Whenever the party's over.

20. If I could sum up my beauty routine simply, I would say it's:
A. Sensible.
(B.) Practical.
C. Time-consuming.

I do what I have to and that's it.

Jose says:
Jamie Lee had a terrible problem. Her hair had no pizzazz whatsoever. For many years her wonderful face was hidden by hair. So we cut it very short, in a way that very few people can wear, and it changed her life. Now she is much more aware of her beautiful face and she has a look that is special.

Andrea Eastman

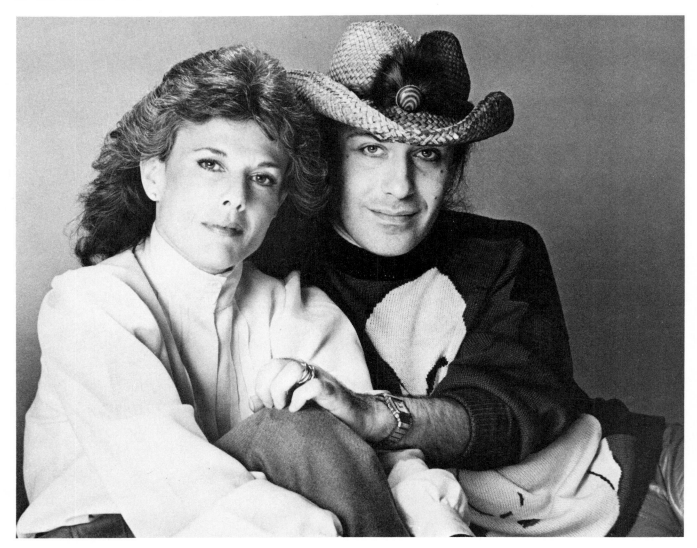

Andrea Eastman is the personal manager for many stars, and I have known her for a long
time. She handles Ali MacGraw, Katharine Ross, Stockard Channing, Jan Michael Vincent,
Hart Bochner, and Jamie Lee Curtis. Andrea came out of Life-style Red, but she could very well
be Life-style Green also. She is a working woman who only has time for beauty once a day
and has to look good for a long time. But because she rides her horses every day, she has a
very sportive side that has to be considered in her daily routine, and that makes her more
Red than Green.

   Married, with her step-children away in college, Andrea lives in Malibu, near some of her
famous clients. She and her husband get up early every morning and have breakfast
together. Then, while her husband gets ready for work, Andrea rides and grooms her horses.
Then she comes back to the house, showers, and gets ready for work. Her whole morning
beauty routine takes forty-five minutes. The rest of the morning she works at home, on the
telephone. Then she drives to a lunch date, which may be in Beverly Hills or Hollywood—an
hour's drive from her house. After lunch, she goes to her office and works until 7:00 P.M.
Then she and her husband may meet for dinner or go to a business dinner together. That's
what I call a very long day. And to make up for all this running around during the week,
Andrea stays home all day Friday, Saturday, and Sunday, when her life totally revolves
around her husband, her home, and her horses. Try to come up with the right hairstyle for a
woman with this diverse a life-style! The obvious answer is the hairstyle that will wash and
wear. And Andrea must have agreed with me, because she tested Life-style Red.

JOSE EBER'S LIFE-STYLE QUIZ

Andrea Eastman

1. When I wake up in the morning:

A. I look at the alarm clock and panic. I'm already late.

(B.) Who needs an alarm clock? I'm up with the birds, or the kids, and ready to go.

C. I roll over and go back to sleep for another half hour because last night really was a bit too much.

2. My regular morning routine:

A. Takes no more than half an hour because I'm so busy.

(B.) Is postponed until later in the day, because I'm out the door for tennis or carpool.

C. *I'm real slow in the mornings but once I get moving double speed!* Depend on what I'm doing during the day and what's cooking for the upcoming evening.

3. When I look in the mirror each morning I:

A. Wish I had time to do something about what I see.

(B.) Splash cold water on my face and check the condition of my skin.

C. Study each line, blemish, and soft spot mercilessly, until I'm satisfied I know exactly how to best care for what I've seen.

4. First thing in the morning, my hair:

A. Needs a wash and blow-dry.

(B.) Kind of falls into place, because my haircut is easy to care for.

C. Is almost perfect, because I just had it done yesterday.

5. My hair:

A. Gets cut whenever I'm in the mood or can't do a thing with it.

(B.) Needs to be cut every four–six weeks; otherwise it's unmanageable.

C. Is long to allow me to manage a variety of hairstyles depending on my needs so I just make sure the ends are trimmed frequently.

6. My hair color:

A. Is something I've experimented with myself.

(B.) Yuck! Ruin my hair with chemicals!

C. Is done at the beauty shop every six years. *I had my hair colored seven years ago. It was the worst! I like my gray hair.*

7. The colors I wear most frequently are:

(A.) Neutrals that mix well in the business world: navy, burgundy, cream, and things that are "safe."

B. Bright colors, I love 'em.

C. Whatever the fashion mavens say is "in," as long as it's also flattering to my skin tones.

8. For a purse, I usually carry:

(A.) One good all-purpose bag that goes with all my clothes.

B. Something fun and inexpensive that holds all the junk I carry around.

C. Whatever matches my clothes.

9. The hair appliances I rely on include:

(A.) A round brush and blow-dryer.

B. I have all kinds of stuff, but I never use it.

C. Electric rollers, hairpins, combs, clips, curling iron, crimper, dryers, and brushes.

55

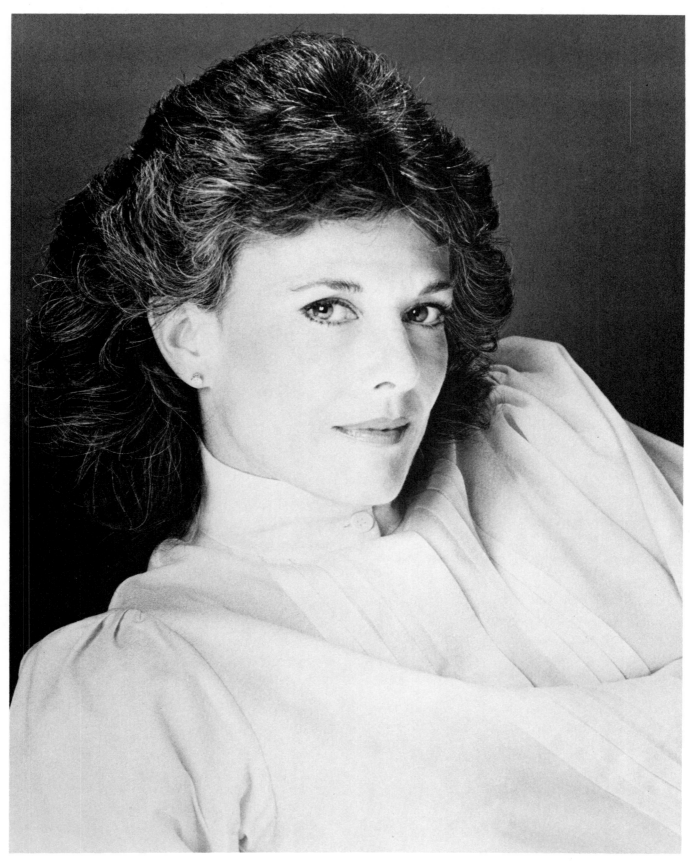

10. **For breakfast, I:**
    A. Grab something on the way to work or eat at my desk
    B. Have cold cereal and fruit.
    (C.) Eat a light meal if I'm dieting or a little more if I'm having a late lunch.

11. **When I bathe, I:**
    (A.) Take a shower first thing in the morning.
    B. Take a shower several times a day, after tennis or swimming.
    C. Take a leisurely bath.

12. **I have help in my home:**
    A. Never.
    B. Once or twice a week.
    (C.) Full time.

13. **I put myself together:**
    (A.) To please myself.
    B. To suit my life-style.
    C. To please my man.

    all three.

14. **I work:**
    A. Nine to five at a regular job.
    B. You think taking care of the kids isn't full-time work?
    C. Flexible hours or not at all.

15. **My fingernails:**
    A. Are manicured by me.

    (B.) Are kept short and neat for simplicity.
    C. I have done weekly.

    Because I ride horses every day.

16. **When it comes to athletics:**
    A. Weekends are the only time I have for recreational sports.
    (B.) I'd only be more active if I were training for the Olympics.
    C. I don't sweat.

17. **If I have a little extra money to splurge with, I:**
    A. Buy something I need.
    (B.) Get something for the kids.
    C. Buy something wonderful I've been dying to have.

    all three reasons.

18. **My idea of the perfect vacation would be to:**
    (A.) Travel to the major cities of Europe.
    B. Go hiking and backpacking.
    C. Glamour it as a bar.

    I'd really prefer a beautiful place south of France, where I could go to nice restaurants and drive around the countryside.

19. **My bedtime is:**
    (A.) After the 11:00 P.M. news.
    B. Early, after an exhausting day.
    C. Whenever the party's over.

20. **If I could sum up my beauty routine simply, I would say it's:**
    A. Sensible.
    (B.) Practical.
    C. Time-consuming.

Jose says:
Andrea has lots and lots of naturally curly hair and a small face, so she feels best when it's cut short enough to have shape. The top is short, because Andrea's face has a tendency to be long-ish, so she doesn't need more length. The full neckline and layers on the side balance her face. This is a wash-and-wear style that is actually cut into her hair. It takes less than five minutes for Andrea to do her hair, which fits her busy life-style.

Farrah Fawcett

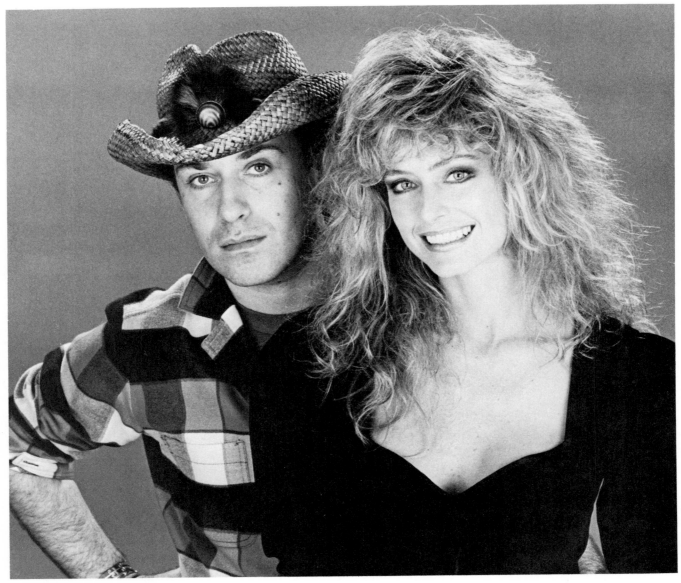

I had an established hairstyle—you know, the Farrah look—but I really wanted a change, and I was doing a series, so I talked to my girl friend Susie Coehlo, and she said to go to Jose. I already knew exactly what I wanted—layer-cut, not length-cut, and someone who respected my natural curl. When I talked with Jose, he said everything that I had felt about my hair. I knew within five minutes that this was my hairdresser.

He never fights me about my hair. He may take what I say and expand on it. We've been together for over six years, and we've done an awful lot of styles. We've made some mistakes and we've had some happy experiences. Sometimes we stop and look at old pictures and start to laugh: we can't believe we did that—what were we thinking of?

I was given a lot of hair and a small face, and when I lose weight, I lose it first in my face. I have a theory that you should use what you have, what God gave you, and take it one step further, not go in the opposite direction or try to be something you're not. I think the Grace Kelly look, with every hair in place, is lovely, but that's not my look. I have a lot of hair, and I like it kind of messy.

I take a sauna every day and some people take that time to sit and read—what else can you do in a sauna? they think. But instead I condition my hair and my nails and my body so I don't dry out too much. It takes half an hour each morning, but then I'm set for the day.

JOSE EBER'S LIFE-STYLE QUIZ   *Farrah Fawcett*

1. When I wake up in the morning:
- **A.** I look at the alarm clock and panic. I'm already late.
- **B.** Who needs an alarm clock? I'm up with the birds, or the kids, and raring to go.
- **C.** I roll over and go back to sleep for another half hour because last night really was a bit too much.

D. I wake up earlier than I have to so I can go back to sleep. I think it comes from doing a series and having to get up at four-thirty in the morning.

2. My regular morning routine:
- **A.** Takes no more than half an hour because I'm so busy.
- (**B.**) Is postponed until later in the day, because I'm out the door for tennis or carpool.
- **C.** Depends on what I'm doing during the day and what's cooking for the upcoming evening.

I have to exercise first.

3. When I look in the mirror each morning I:
- **A.** Wish I had time to do something about what I see.
- (**B.**) Splash cold water on my face and check the condition of my skin.
- **C.** Study each line, blemish, and soft spot mercilessly, until I'm satisfied I know exactly how to best care for what I've seen.

D. When I look in the mirror I can tell what I ate for dinner the night before.

4. First thing in the morning, my hair:
- **A.** Needs a wash and blow-dry.
- (**B.**) Kind of falls into place, because my haircut is easy to care for.
- **C.** Is almost perfect, because I just had it done yesterday.

I really couldn't go out. I just push my hair around until it's big and wild.

5. My hair:
- **A.** Gets cut whenever I'm in the mood or can't do a thing with it.
- **B.** Needs to be cut every four–six weeks; otherwise it's unmanageable.
- **C.** Is long to allow me to manage a variety of hairstyles depending on my needs so I just make sure the ends are trimmed frequently.

It's all three. It gets cut every six weeks, I'd say.

6. My hair color:
- **A.** Is something I've experimented with myself.
- **B.** Yuck! Ruin my hair with chemicals?
- (**C.**) Is done at the beauty shop every six weeks.

D. Is done at the beauty shop, irregularly, actually, with a lot of help from the sun and some lemons.

7. The colors I wear most frequently are:
- **A.** Neutrals that mix well in the business world: navy, burgundy, cream, and things that are "safe."
- **B.** Bright colors, I love 'em.
- **C.** Whatever the fashion mavens say is "in," as long as it's also flattering to my skin tones.

D. It depends on my mood, they may be old clothes or new clothes or neutrals or bright colors.

8. For a purse, I usually carry:
- **A.** One good all-purpose bag that goes with all my clothes.
- **B.** Something fun and inexpensive that holds all the junk I carry around.
- **C.** Whatever matches my clothes.

D. One big leather pouch I've had for years that holds everything.

9. The hair appliances I rely on include:
- **A.** A round brush and blow-dryer.
- **B.** I have all kinds of stuff, but I never use it.
- (**C.**) Electric rollers, hairpins, combs, clips, curling iron, crimper, dryers, and brushes.

59

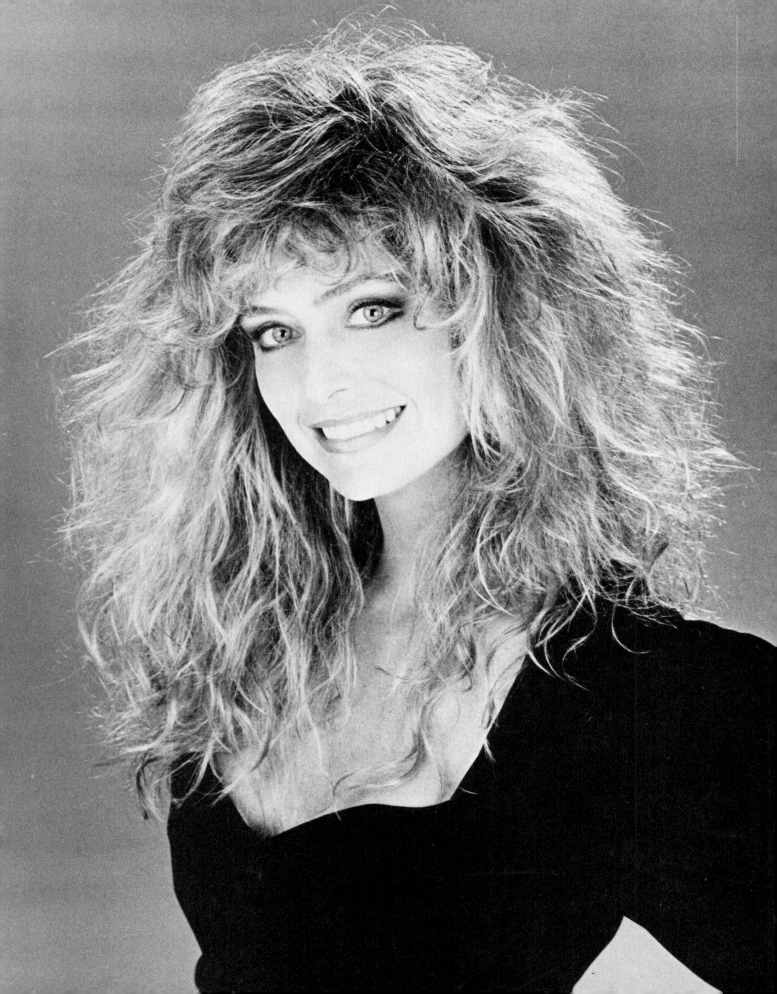

10. **For breakfast, I:**
    A. Grab something on the way to work or eat at my desk
    B. Have cold cereal and fruit.
    C. Eat a light meal if I'm dieting or a little more if I'm having a late lunch.

    D. I have a cup of tea.

11. **When I bathe, I:**
    A. Take a shower first thing in the morning.
    (B.) Take a shower several times a day, after tennis or swimming.
    C. Take a leisurely bath.

    I take a sauna play racquetball then I have a jacuzzi at night; I count that as a bath.

12. **I have help in my home:**
    A. Never.
    B. Once or twice a week.
    (C.) Full time.

    always. I figure, just go for it.

13. **I put myself together:**
    A. To please myself.
    B. To suit my life-style.
    C. To please my man.

    all three

14. **I work:**
    A. Nine to five at a regular job.
    B. You think taking care of the kids isn't full-time work?
    C. Flexible hours or not at all.

15. **My fingernails:**
    A. Are manicured by me.

    (B.) Are kept short and neat for simplicity.
    C. I hate them.

    I do them myself but I keep them short.

16. **When it comes to athletics:**
    A. Weekends are the only time I have for recreational sports.
    (B.) I'd only be more active if I were training for the Olympics.
    C. I don't sweat.

17. **If I have a little extra money to splurge with, I:**
    A. Buy something I need.
    (B.) Get something for the kids.
    C. Buy something wonderful I've been dying to have.

18. **My idea of the perfect vacation would be to:**
    (A.) Travel to the major cities of Europe.
    B. Go hiking and backpacking.
    C. Escape to a spa.

19. **My bedtime is:**
    A. After the 11:00 P.M. news.
    B. Early, after an exhausting day.
    C. Whenever the party's over.

    All of them. It may be 11:30; it may be 2:30.

20. **If I could sum up my beauty routine simply, I would say it's:**
    A. Sensible.
    B. Practical.
    C. Time-consuming.

    D. I call it being on the go. I'm always running out of the house and finishing my beauty routine in the car!

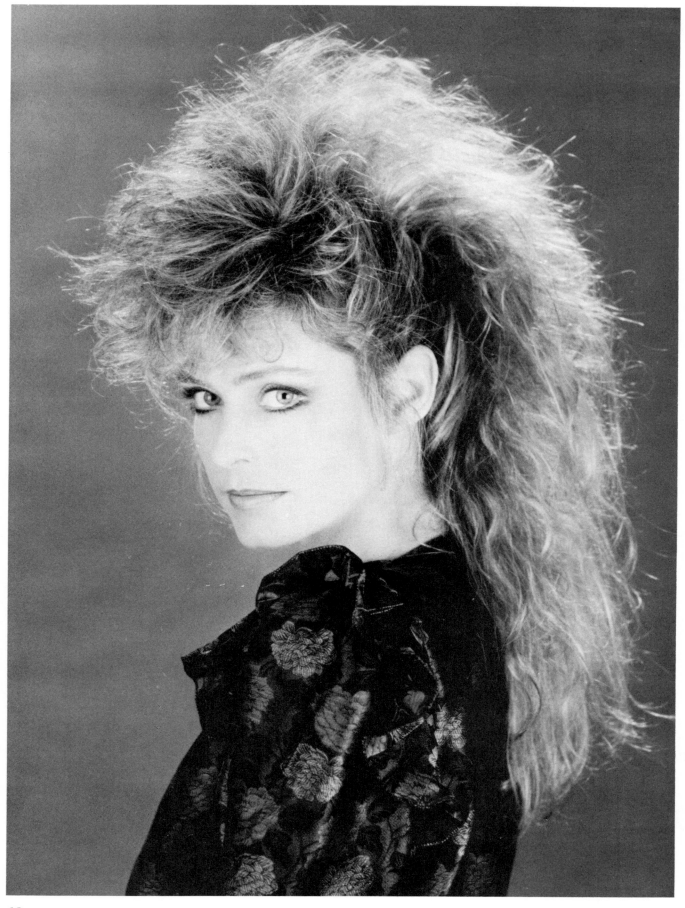

Jose says:

Because it's naturally wavy, Farrah has the ideal hair that every woman wants. She can do anything with it; she just feels sexier with long hair. Her hair is always layered, to let the natural curl do whatever it wants. She can wash her hair and finger-style it—she needs no brush or hair dryer—and all you see is tons of hair, wonderful hair.

Every now and then, you just get tired of the way you look; this happens to everyone. You want to do something that is fun, maybe even silly, even if it isn't practical or the kind of hairstyle you could wear to the office or to the market or in your real world life. So I call this a fantasy look.

Farrah and I have a lot of fun with fantasy looks because often we work together in photo lay-outs where we can let our imaginations run free and do whatever wild and crazy things we think of at the time. Sometimes we look back at these pictures and poke each other's sides and ask if we were nuts or something. But these hairstyles are just done for a look. They are only for the moment. Sometimes they don't even make sense a week later. They depend on mood, a need for adventure, a craving to be different. Sometimes these fantasy styles are even chosen for their shock value.

So here you see two pictures of Farrah. One is a regular picture. She looks very good, no? The other is the fantasy picture. I think she looks fantastic! We call this The Mohawk and we love it because it dares to be different, to be fun, to be bold, to be startlingly new. It is not for everyone!

Ali MacGraw

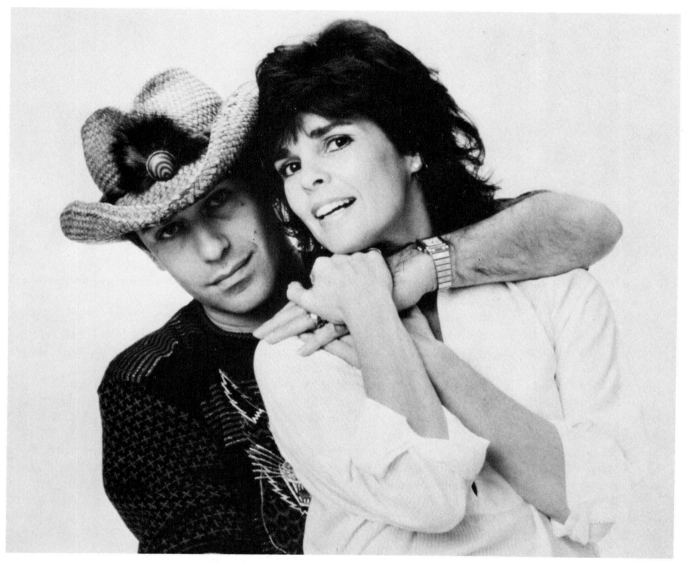

I met Jose about five years ago when I had taken it upon myself to cut all my hair off. After the amusement of this adventure wore off, I had a fit of self-loathing when I faced the fact that I was going to look awful for three years until my hair grew out, so I decided to get professional hair help immediately. I went to Jose and said "help" and he looked at me with true horror and incredulity. I felt the most hideous I have ever felt in my whole life.

Jose took me under his wing and finally I got healthy hair. I'm passed the time in my life where I want to make a fashion statement. I wouldn't do a punk hairstyle just because I thought it was amusing. I never think of hair in terms of face shape. I just think hair should look like it would be nice to touch it—except on stage of course. And it's important sexually speaking. A man wants touchable hair, I think.

I live at the beach and I like a real informal kind of life. I use a conditioner that friends bring me from Germany. It smells like lemon souffle. I use henna for body, not color. I despise red henna. My hair is in great condition because of Araxy's magic potions and my hair has a good cut because of Jose.

JOSE EBER'S LIFE-STYLE QUIZ *Ali MacGraw*

1. When I wake up in the morning:

  A. I look at the alarm clock and panic. I'm already late.

  B. Who needs an alarm clock? I'm up with the birds, or the kids, and ready to go.

  C. I roll over and go back to sleep for another half hour because last night really was a bit too much.

  D. I get right out of bed, never looking back.

2. My regular morning routine:

  (A.) Takes no more than half an hour because I'm so busy.

  B. Is postponed until later in the day, because I'm out the door for tennis or carpool.

  C. Depends on what I'm doing during the day and what's cooking for the upcoming evening.

3. When I look in the mirror each morning I:

  A. Wish I had time to do something about what I see.

  B. Splash cold water on my face and check the condition of my skin.

  C. Study each line, element, and stuff mercilessly until I'm satisfied I know exactly how to best care for what I've gotten.

  D. I get into the shower and do a dance under that water and then stretches and I wash my hair in rinse myself in an ice cold shower.

4. First thing in the morning, my hair:

  A. Needs a wash and blow-dry.

  B. Kind of falls into place, because my haircut is easy to care for.

  C. Is almost perfect, because I just had it cut yesterday.

  D. My hair washes make do with cold water or some shampoos and a shake dry.

5. My hair:

  A. Gets cut whenever I'm in the mood or can't do a thing with it.

  (B.) Needs to be cut every four–six weeks; otherwise it's unmanageable.

  C. Is long to allow me to manage a variety of hairstyles depending on my needs so I just make sure the ends are trimmed frequently.

6. My hair color:

  A. Is something I've experimented with myself.

  B. Yuck! Ruin my hair with chemicals?

  (C.) Is done at the beauty shop every six weeks *when I'm working.*

7. The colors I wear most frequently are:

  A. Neutrals that mix well in the business world: navy, burgundy, cream, and things that are "safe."

  B. Bright colors I love 'em.

  C. Whatever the fashion mavens say is "in," as long as it's also flattering to my skin tones.

  D. I like black and white and red.

8. For a purse, I usually carry:

  A. One good all-purpose bag that goes with all my clothes.

  B. Something fun and inexpensive that I don't mind if I junk carry around.

  D. **C.** Whatever matches my clothes.

  D. I carry whatever I feel like; it may be expensive one day and not the next. It all depends on what I'm wearing, and changing my handbag just to be matchy-matchy.

9. The hair appliances I rely on include:

  A. A round brush and blow-dryer.

  B. I have all kinds of stuff, but I never use it.

  C. Electric rollers, hairpins, combs, clips, curling iron, trimmer, dryers, and brushes.

  D. Great shampoo and conditioner. That's it.

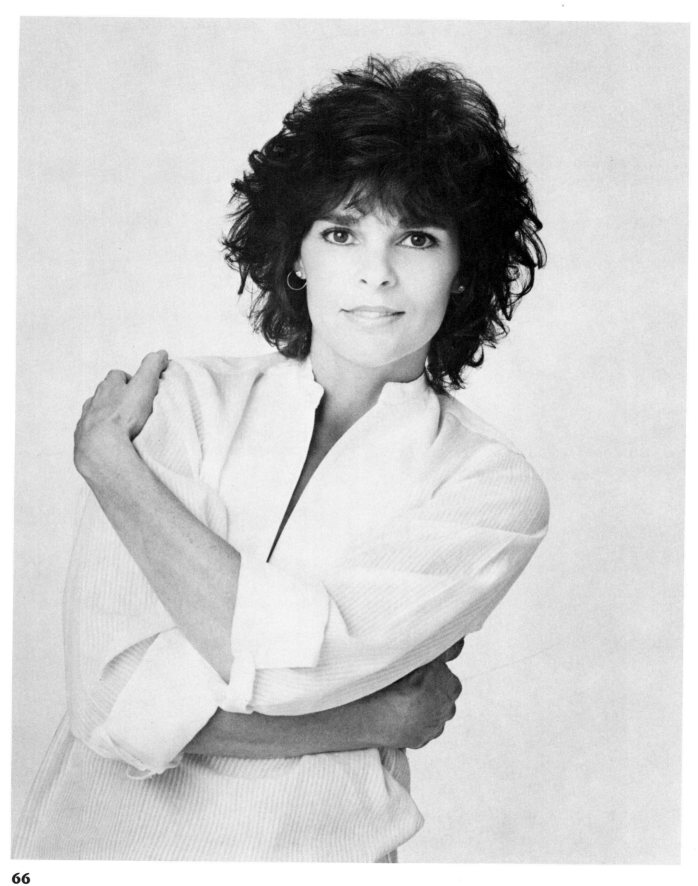

10. **For breakfast, I:**
    A. Grab something on the way to work, or eat at my desk.
    B. Have cold cereal and fruit.
    C. Eat a light meal if I'm dieting, or a little more if I'm having a late lunch.

    For breakfast I have lemon juice, decaffeinated coffee with honey, and grain bread with honey on everything.

11. **When I bathe, I:**
    A. Take a shower first thing in the morning.
    B. Take a shower several times a day, after tennis or swimming.
    C. Take a leisurely bath.

    D. Shower every morning, bathe at night.

12. **I have help in my home:**
    A. Never.
    B. Once or twice a week.
    C. Full time.

    whenever I need it, it depends on my work schedule.

13. **I put myself together:**
    A. To please myself. *(circled)*
    B. To suit my life-style.
    C. To please my man.

    in a way that makes me feel totally comfortable with myself and that's usually what makes a man feel good.

14. **I work:**
    A. Nine to five at a regular job.
    B. You think taking care of the kids isn't full-time work?
    C. Flexible hours or not at all.

15. **My fingernails:**
    A. Are manicured by me.
    B. Are kept short and neat for simplicity.
    C. I have done weekly. *(circled)*

16. **When it comes to athletics:**
    A. Weekends are the only time I have for recreational sports.
    B. I'd only be more active if I were training for the Olympics.
    C. I don't sweat.

    I'm terrible so unathletic as often as possible.

17. **If I have a little extra money to splurge with, I:**
    A. Buy something I need.
    B. Get something for the kids.
    C. Buy something wonderful I've been dying to have.

    D. Buy more flowers.

18. **My idea of the perfect vacation would be to:**
    A. Travel to the major cities of Europe.
    B. Go hiking and backpacking.
    C. Escape to a spa.

    I like to have adventure. I've never it could be three. I love backpacking to any of these. Maybe I'd go to a spa or to Paris or Venice.

19. **My bedtime is:**
    A. After the 11:00 P.M. news.
    B. Early, after an exhausting day.
    C. Whenever the party's over.

    D. Wildly variable.

20. **If I could sum up my beauty routine simply, I would say it's:**
    A. Sensible.
    B. Practical.
    C. Time consuming.

    my beauty look is at its best when I'm rested, healthy, and happy. Red! That's me. Isn't everybody?

Jose says:

Ali is a natural type who doesn't want to fool around with her hair. She lives at the beach and wants her hairstyle to be easy, so she has short layers, for a wash-and-wear style that is ideal for her. But there is enough length to her hair that she can look glamourous when she has to. She has enough hair to use electric rollers or a curling iron for something special. But she is a funky, carefree kind of person, and her hairstyle has to match her life-style.

Melissa Manchester

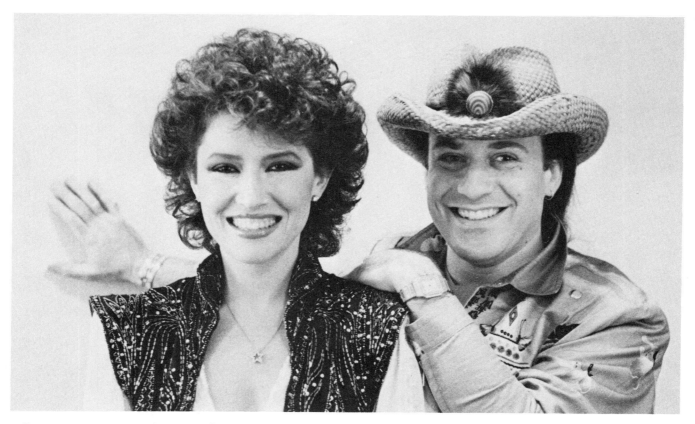

I first met Jose at a shooting for a record album. It was the first time I'd used him, the photographer, Steve Schapiro, and Wayne Masserelli, the makeup artist, and we all clicked. We all got together to recreate a photograph that George Hurrell had taken of Katharine Hepburn in the forties. My hair was much longer then, and it's very thick. Jose did my hair, and from that time on I knew he was right for me. Now he does my hair whenever I need a cut or when I do pictures or concerts or a television appearance. Beyond a certain point, I don't know anything about hair at all. I can take care of it myself for every day, but for special occasions I need Jose. I sweat a lot on stage, especially when my hair is long and it flies around.

Instead of trying to straighten my hair into a pageboy, Jose made the thick curls work for me. Cutting it short was his idea, and now I'm growing it again, and that was his idea, too. I was doing a Bob Hope special, and I wore a tuxedo, so Jose pinned my hair up and he said to me, "Darling, the next time, I am going to cut your hair." So he did. It was summer then, and it felt really great. Then, a few weeks ago, Jose said, "Enough of the short hair, darling; let's do something different." So we're keeping it short on the top and letting the back grow longer. I'm trying to look like Jackie Bisset.

I have very curly hair, so I blow it dry to untighten the curl. When it grows out, it grows sideways instead of down, so I have to be careful not to look like a pyramid. I need a good conditioner and a good cut.

When I was growing up, I wanted straight hair so badly, I even tried to iron it. When curly hair came into fashion, I was thrilled. But I'm not a beauty-parlor person, so I don't go in too much for fads or looks. I've never thought I had to have the style everyone else had, just because it was in. But I'm thinking about having a Mohawk . . . I'm just kidding. My hair has its own personality. It's thick and it's curly, so it creates its own persona, and it's the dominant aspect of my look. I guess you'd call it the wild-and-woolly look.

But it's easy to care for and easy to style. I can do a lot of things with combs and accessories, and I like hats a lot. In fifteen minutes I can blow it straight or have it frizzy. I guess I have what some women try to get with a permanent. But it's all natural on me, baby.

JOSE EBER'S LIFE-STYLE QUIZ   *Melissa Manchester*

1. **When I wake up in the morning:**
   A. I look at the alarm clock and panic. I'm already late.
   B. (circled) Who needs an alarm clock? I'm up with the birds, or the kids, and ready to go.
   C. I roll over and go back to sleep for another half hour because last night really was a bit too much.

2. **My regular morning routine:**
   A. Takes no more than half an hour because I'm so busy.
   B. Is postponed until later in the day, because I'm out the door for tennis or carpool.
   C. (circled) Depends on what I'm doing during the day and what's cooking for the upcoming evening.

3. **When I look in the mirror each morning I:**
   A. Wish I had time to do something about what I see.
   B. (circled) Splash cold water on my face and check the condition of my skin.
   C. Study each line, blemish, and soft spot meticulously, until I'm satisfied I know exactly how to best care for what I've seen.
   and I don't pick at the bridge, or open the pores after?

4. **First thing in the morning, my hair:**
   A. (circled) Needs a wash and blow-dry.
   B. Kind of falls into place, because my haircut is easy to care for.
   C. Is almost perfect, because I just had it done yesterday.

5. **My hair:**
   A. Gets cut whenever I'm in the mood or can't do a thing with it.
   B. (circled) Needs to be cut every four–six weeks; otherwise it's unmanageable.
   C. Is long to allow me to manage a variety of hairstyles depending on my needs so I just make sure the ends are trimmed frequently.

6. **My hair color:**
   A. Is something I've experimented with myself.
   B. (circled) Yuck! Ruin my hair with chemicals?
   C. Is done at the beauty shop every six weeks.
   I like to keep my two gray hairs right in place.

7. **The colors I wear most frequently are:**
   A. Neutrals that mix well in the business world: navy, burgundy, cream, and things that are "safe."
   B. (circled) Bright colors, I love 'em.
   C. Whatever the fashion mavens say is "in," as long as it's also flattering to my skin tones.

8. **For a purse, I usually carry:**
   A. (circled) One good all-purpose bag that goes with all my clothes.
   B. Something fun and inexpensive that holds all the junk I carry around.
   C. Whatever matches my clothes.
   all three.

9. **The hair appliances I rely on include:**
   A. (circled) A round brush and blow-dryer.
   B. I have all kinds of stuff, but I never use it.
   C. Electric rollers, hairpins, combs, clips, curling iron, crimper, dryers, and brushes.

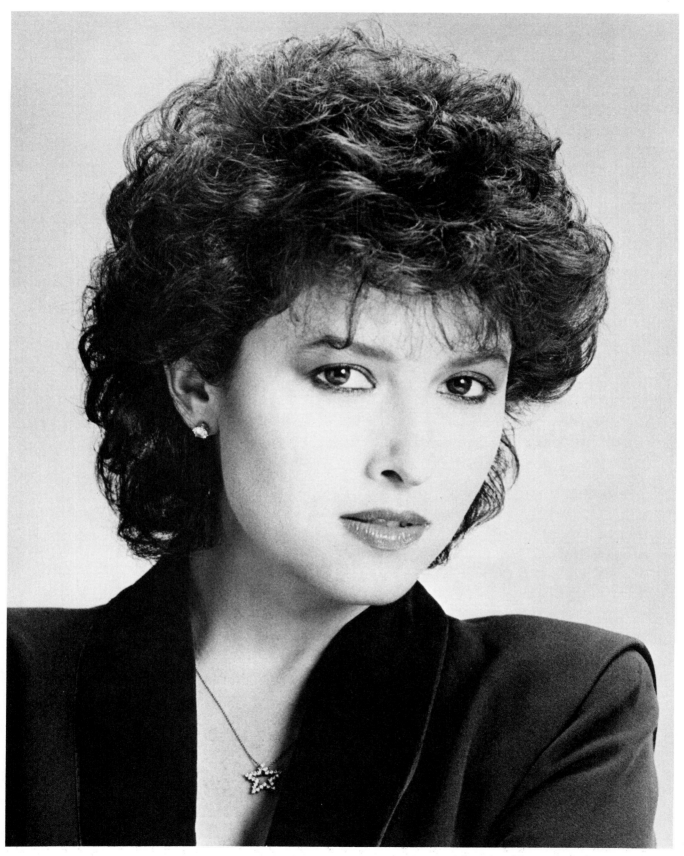

Melissa's makeup by Wayne Masserelli.

10. **For breakfast, I:**
    A. Grab something on the way to work or eat at my desk
    B. Have cold cereal and fruit.
    C. Eat a light meal if I'm dieting or a little more if I'm having a late lunch.

11. **When I bathe, I:**
    A. Take a shower first thing in the morning.
    B. Take a shower several times a day, after tennis or swimming.
    C. Take a leisurely bath.

12. **I have help in my home:**
    A. Never.
    B. Once or twice a week.
    C. Full time.

13. **I put myself together:**
    A. To please myself.
    B. To suit my life-style.
    C. To please my man.

14. **I work:**
    A. Nine to five at a regular job.
    B. You think taking care of the kids isn't full-time work?
    C. Flexible hours or not at all.

15. **My fingernails:**
    A. Are manicured by me.
    B. Are kept short and neat for simplicity.
    C. I have done weekly.

16. **When it comes to athletics:**
    A. Weekends are the only time I have for recreational sports.
    B. I'd only be more active if I were training for the Olympics.
    C. I don't sweat.

17. **If I have a little extra money to splurge with, I:**
    A. Buy something I need.
    B. Get something for the kids.
    C. Buy something wonderful I've been dying to have.

18. **My idea of the perfect vacation would be to:**
    A. Travel to the major cities of Europe.
    B. Go hiking and backpacking.
    C. Escape to a spa.

19. **My bedtime is:**
    A. After the 11:00 P.M. news.
    B. Early, after an exhausting day.
    C. Whenever the party's over.

    It's A unless there's a good movie on TV.

20. **If I could sum up my beauty routine simply, I would say it's:**
    A. Sensible.
    B. Practical.
    C. Time-consuming.

Jose says:
Now Melissa has short hair, but sometimes she lets it grow. Either way, with her hair, the idea is to let it do what it wants, because of the natural curl, and to control it so she doesn't look like a bush. Since her face is small, we don't want lots of wild hair covering it. That's why there are layers cut into the top part of her hair, for a little height. This keeps the hair up and off her face and back at the temples.

Penny Marshall

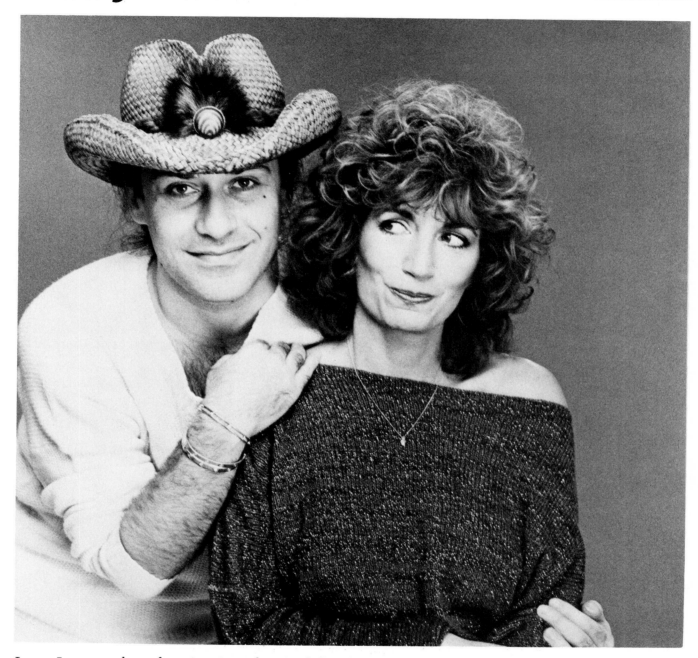

I met Jose one day when Carrie Fisher said, "Let's go get our hair cut at Jose's." I had had my hair cut in France, when I thought I was asking how to find a masseuse and ended up with a haircut. Jose spoke French, so I thought it was all the same thing. He cut my hair, and he did it right.

He kept saying I have great hair, which is news to me. It's only great when he does it and for two days after. When we're left alone, my hair and I don't get along.

I have naturally curly hair, and now it's cut to go with the curl. Jose said that was very important. So I wash my hair in the shower and use whatever creme rinse is around and get out of the shower. I'm supposed to squeeze my hair in place and blow it around with the dryer a little bit, but my arm gets tired.

I actually wish I had hair like Jose's, with a long braid down my back, but I don't look good with my hair pulled back from my face. In fact, I like to have a lot of hair around my face, maybe even to hide my face.

JOSE EBER'S LIFE-STYLE QUIZ   *Penny Marshall*

1. When I wake up in the morning:
A. I look at the alarm clock and panic. I'm already late.
B. Who needs an alarm clock? I'm up with the birds, or the kids, and ready to go.
C. I roll over and go back to sleep for another half hour because last night really was a bit too much.

D. I get up because I [called] then I lie in bed for fifteen minutes before I [get up] in a stupor... run for my life.

2. My regular morning routine:
(A.) Takes no more than half an hour because I'm so busy.
B. Is postponed until later in the day, because I'm out the door for tennis or carpool.
C. Depends on what I'm doing during the day and what so looking for the upcoming evening.

It's not quite a routine.

3. When I look in the mirror each morning I:
A. Wish I had time to do something about what I see.
B. Splash cold water on my face and check the condition of my skin.
C. Study each line, blemish and soft spot mercilessly, until I'm satisfied I know exactly how to best go for what I've seen.

D. I don't look in the mirror in the morning that would be horrifying.

4. First thing in the morning, my hair:
A. Needs a wash and blow-dry.
B. Kind of falls into place, because my haircut is easy to care for.
C. Is almost perfect because I just had it done yesterday.

D. I shower and does whatever it does.

5. My hair:
A. Gets cut whenever I'm in the mood or can't do a thing with it.
B. Needs to be cut every four–six weeks otherwise it's unmanageable.
C. Is long to allow me to manage a variety of hairstyles depending on my needs so I just make sure the ends are trimmed frequently.

D. When somebody [says], "you need a haircut," I get one.

6. My hair color:
A. Is something I've experimented with myself.
B. Yuck! Ruin my hair with chemicals?
C. Is done at the beauty shop every six weeks.

D. When somebody says "You need your hair highlighted," I get it done.

7. The colors I wear most frequently are:
A. Neutrals that mix well in the business world: navy, burgundy, cream, and things that are "safe."
B. Bright colors, I love 'em.
C. Whatever the fashion mavens say is "in," as long as it's also flattering to my skin tones.

D. Denim

8. For a purse, I usually carry:
A. One good all-purpose bag that goes with all my clothes.
B. Something fun and inexpensive that holds all the junk I carry around.
C. Whatever matches my clothes.

D. [It's not important. I tend to much into whether expensive or inexpensive.]

9. The hair appliances I rely on include:
A. A round brush and blow-dryer.
B. I have all kinds of stuff, but I never use it.
C. Electric rollers, hairpins, combs, clips, curling iron, crimper, dryers, and brushes.

73

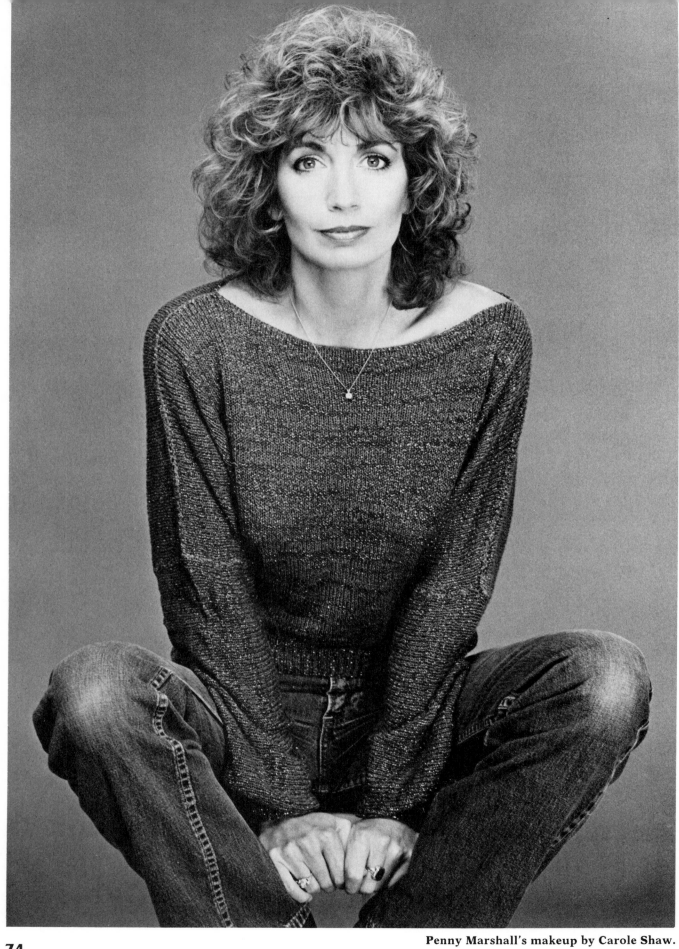

Penny Marshall's makeup by Carole Shaw.

10. **For breakfast, I:**
    A. Grab something on the way to work or eat at my desk
    B. Have cold cereal and fruit.
    C. Eat a light meal if I'm dieting or a little more if I'm having a late lunch.
    D. I drink coffee.

11. **When I bathe, I:**
    A. Take a shower first thing in the morning.
    (B.) Take a shower several times a day, after tennis or swimming.
    C. Take a leisurely bath.
    all three, but I'm not into sports.

12. **I have help in my home:**
    A. Never.
    B. Once or twice a week.
    C. Full time.
    D. It depends on where I'm living and whether it comes with the house.

13. **I put myself together:**
    A. To please myself.
    B. To suit my life-style.
    C. To please my man.
    D. I never quite put it together.

14. **I work:**
    A. Nine to five at a regular job.
    B. You think taking care of the kids isn't full-time work?
    C. Flexible hours or not at all.

15. **My fingernails:**
    A. Are manicured by me.
    B. Are kept short and neat for simplicity.
    C. I have done mostly by the
    D. I bite them to the point of neurosis.

16. **When it comes to athletics:**
    A. Weekends are the only time I have for recreational sports.
    B. I'd only be more productive if I were training at the Olympics.
    C. I don't sweat.
    D. I sweat but I don't like athletics

17. **If I have a little extra money to splurge with, I:**
    A. Buy something I need.
    B. Get something for the kids.
    C. Buy something wonderful I've been dying to have.
    D. It's never happened

18. **My idea of the perfect vacation would be to:**
    A. Travel to the major cities of Europe.
    B. Go hiking and backpacking.
    C. Escape to a spa.
    D. Travel the minor cities of Europe.

19. **My bedtime is:**
    A. After the 11:00 P.M. news.
    B. Early, after an exhausting day.
    C. Whatever time the party's over.
    D. I have trouble sleeping—who knows when my bedtime is?

20. **If I could sum up my beauty routine simply, I would say it's:**
    A. Sensible.
    B. Practical.
    C. Time-consuming.
    D. Nonexistent

Jose says:
Penny has wonderful naturally curly hair, and its texture is light and fluffy, so she can have a carefree-looking hairstyle that is easy to do, which is what she likes. She has bangs, and then the hair is layered all over to allow the curl to do what it wants. The cut merely follows the curl. Then Penny lets it go, and it's wonderful. The cut frames the face and gives her the funky, messy look that makes her feel comfortable, but with a blow-dryer or hot rollers she can have any style.

Valerie Perrine

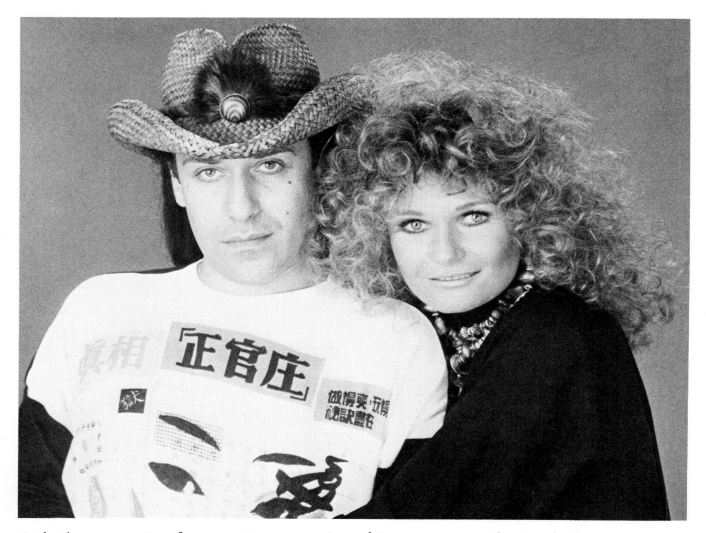

Gosh, I've gone to Jose for years. Let me see, I met him at a party at Alan Carr's about two or three years ago. My good girl friend Pat Van Patten introduced us. I knew how famous he was and what a good job he did, so I asked him to do a *Playboy* photo session for me. He did my hair in a way I'd never seen before, and that was it. We've been together since. But I hardly ever go to the shop. I went there just once, as a matter of fact, when I was so late, I had to stop by on the way to my appointment. Usually Jose comes to my house. And a lot of the time I cut my hair myself, with a manicure scissors. I do a very good job, but Jose gets hysterical.

I don't like my face to look too round, so I'm careful with shadowing on the cheeks. And I like my bangs to have shape and curve around my face, not just to lie straight across my forehead. Sometimes I mess up on them, and then Jose has to fix them.

But I never fool around with the length. I want my hair to grow to my waist. It feels good long when it tickles my back. I love long hair.

JOSE EBER'S LIFE-STYLE QUIZ

Valerie Perrine

1. **When I wake up in the morning:**
   A. I look at the alarm clock and panic. I'm already late.
   B. Who needs an alarm clock? I'm up with the birds, or the kids, and ready to go.
   C. I roll over and go back to sleep for another half hour because last night really was a bit too much.

2. **My regular morning routine:**
   A. Takes no more than half an hour because I'm so busy.
   B. Is postponed until later in the day, because I'm out the door for tennis or carpool.
   C. Depends on what I'm doing during the day and what's cooking for the upcoming evening.

3. **When I look in the mirror each morning I:**
   A. Wish I had time to do something about what I see.
   B. Splash cold water on my face and check the condition of my skin.
   C. Study each line, blemish, and soft spot mercilessly, until I'm satisfied I know exactly how to best care for what I've seen.

4. **First thing in the morning, my hair:**
   A. Needs a wash and blow-dry.
   B. Kind of falls into place, because my haircut is easy to care for.
   C. Is almost perfect, because I just had it done yesterday.

5. **My hair:**
   A. Gets cut whenever I'm in the mood or can't do a thing with it.
   B. Needs to be cut every four–six weeks, otherwise it's unmanageable.
   C. Is long to allow me to manage a variety of hairstyles depending on my needs so I just make sure the ends are trimmed frequently.

   It's sort of but it's really B. I cut my own bangs, then Jose grabs me and says it's time for a cut.

6. **My hair color:**
   A. Is something I've experimented with myself.
   B. Yuck! Ruin my hair with chemicals?
   C. Is done at the beauty shop every six weeks.

   none of these. Oh I guess it's C. I have it done at home; I'm not a beauty parlor person.

7. **The colors I wear most frequently are:**
   A. Neutrals that mix well in the business world: navy, burgundy, cream, and things that are "safe."
   B. Bright colors, I love 'em.
   C. Whatever the fashion mavens say is "in," as long as it's also flattering to my skin tones.

8. **For a purse, I usually carry:**
   A. One good all-purpose bag that goes with all my clothes.
   B. Something fun and inexpensive that holds all the junk I carry around.
   C. Whatever matches my clothes.

9. **The hair appliances I rely on include:**
   A. A round brush and blow-dryer.
   B. I have all kinds of stuff, but I never use it.
   C. Electric rollers, hairpins, combs, clips, curling iron, crimper, dryers, and brushes.

77

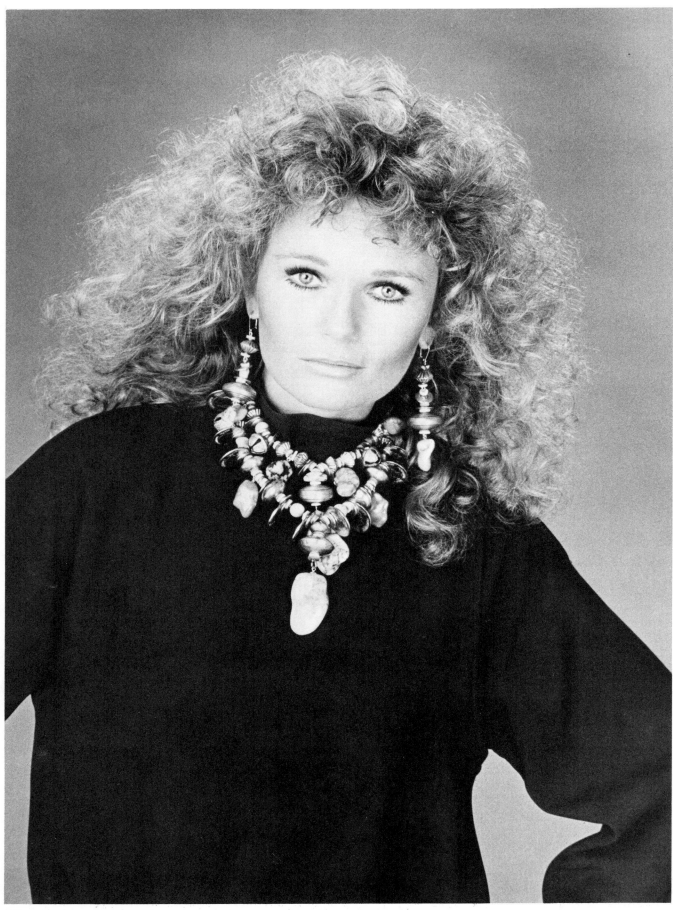

10. **For breakfast, I:**
    A. Grab something on the way to work or eat at my desk
    B. Have cold cereal and fruit.
    C. Eat a light meal if I'm dieting or a little more if I'm having a late lunch.

    I never eat breakfast.

11. **When I bathe, I:**
    A. Take a shower first thing in the morning.
    B. Take a shower several times a day, after tennis or swimming.
    C. Take a leisurely bath.

12. **I have help in my home:**
    A. Never.
    B. Once or twice a week.
    C. Full time.

13. **I put myself together:**
    A. To please myself.
    B. To suit my life-style.
    C. To please my man.

14. **I work:**
    A. Nine to five at a regular job.
    B. You think taking care of the kids isn't full-time work?
    C. Flexible hours or not at all.

15. **My fingernails:**
    A. Are manicured by me.
    B. Are kept short and neat for simplicity.
    C. I have done weekly.

16. **When it comes to athletics:**
    A. Weekends are the only time I have for recreational sports.
    B. I'd only be more active if I were training for the Olympics.
    C. I don't sweat.

17. **If I have a little extra money to splurge with, I:**
    A. Buy something I need.
    B. Get something for the kids.
    C. Buy something wonderful I've been dying to have.

18. **My idea of the perfect vacation would be to:**
    A. Travel to the major cities of Europe.
    B. Go hiking and backpacking.
    C. Escape to a spa.

    Hmmm, this really depends on my mood.

19. **My bedtime is:**
    A. After the 11:00 P.M. news.
    B. Early, after an exhausting day.
    C. Whenever the party's over.

20. **If I could sum up my beauty routine simply, I would say it's:**
    A. Sensible.
    B. Practical.
    C. Time-consuming.

    Well, it's sensible to be practical, isn't it?

Jose says:
Valerie's hair is baby-fine, so it is not layered; it is cut to give the illusion of being one length. She can wear her hair this way because of her wonderful bone structure, which the cut accentuates. The bangs we cut very wide, to show up her beautiful eyes. Her hair does not need a perm with this style, and we can use curling irons or curlers or tissue papers for waves and curls on special occasions. Valerie's hair is so fine, it is better for her to avoid hot rollers and curling irons so she does not break the ends. Valerie has a face that looks equally good with the hair up or down, and she can wear a lot of different styles because of her bone structure.

Katharine Ross

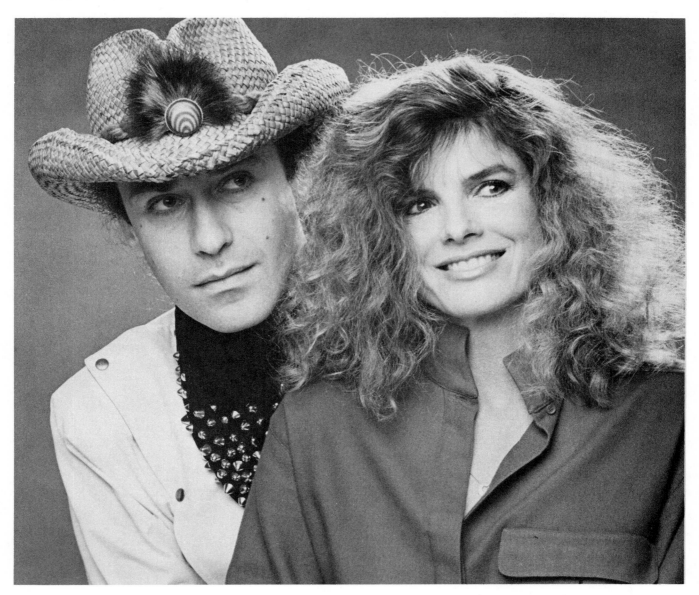

I had very long straight hair that just hung, and I badly needed to have it cut, but I really was terrified, and finally my agent suggested that I go to Jose. I think I went to him for a year and a half before I let him cut off more than an inch. I was basically going to him to get the ends trimmed. He'd say, "Why don't you cut this and that?" and I'd say, "I just can't," and he was very sensitive to that. He always cut off just the amount he said he was going to—no sudden or swift surprises, like some hairstylists give you.

I was working my way toward cutting it off, but it was taking me a while. Finally, I did it. I was nervous, but then immediately thrilled. I knew I hadn't made a mistake. Cutting it had nothing to do with a film or a role; I just did it for myself.

It's really easy to take care of. I shampoo it every other day and try to let it dry naturally, and that's it. I do nothing to it. It used to kind of hang there, with no style. Now I have a perm, and I can just shove my hair under a hat when I run or ride, and then wash it and let it dry, and it looks great. For special occasions, Jose might wrap it in tissue paper and curl it, but I don't normally do that myself. I live at the beach, and I like to be casual.

I don't go much by face shape or any of that stuff for picking a hairstyle; I just like to have hair around my shoulders. I don't want my hair to be too short, because I need versatility. And I'm more comfortable when I have more hair.

JOSE EBER'S LIFE-STYLE QUIZ   *Katharine Ross*

1. When I wake up in the morning:
  A. I look at the alarm clock and panic. I'm already late.
  (B.) Who needs an alarm clock? I'm up with the birds, or the kids, and ready to go.
  C. I roll over and go back to sleep for another half an hour because last night really was a bit too much.

I hope Katharine Ross is not ruled out because I come out red in some foreign languages.

2. My regular morning routine:
  (A.) Takes no more than half an hour because I'm so busy.
  B. Is postponed until later in the day, because I'm out the door for tennis or carpool.
  C. Depends on what I'm doing during the day and what's cooking for the upcoming evening.

3. When I look in the mirror each morning I:
  A. Wish I had time to do something about what I see.
  (B.) Splash cold water on my face and check the condition of my skin.
  C. Study each line, blemish, and soft spot mercilessly, until I'm satisfied I know what my face can best care for what I've given up.

Hmm, well, I know Jack! I get it's true until I get my face up. B is a better answer than the others.

4. First thing in the morning, my hair:
  A. Needs a wash and blow-dry.
  (B.) Kind of falls into place, because my haircut is easy to care for.
  C. Is almost perfect, because I just had it done yesterday.

It's B and C, but more B.

5. My hair:
  (A.) Gets cut whenever I'm in the mood or can't do a thing with it.
  B. Needs to be cut every four–six weeks; otherwise it's unmanageable.
  C. Is long to allow me to manage a variety of hairstyles depending on my needs so I just make sure the ends are trimmed frequently.

A or C. I guess C

6. My hair color:
  A. Is something I've experimented with myself.
  B. Yuck! Ruin my hair with chemicals?
  C. Is done at the beauty shop every six weeks.

None of the above.

7. The colors I wear most frequently are:
  A. Neutrals that mix well in the business world: navy, burgundy, cream, and things that are "safe."
  (B.) Bright colors. I love them.
  C. Whatever the fashion mavens say is "in" as long as it's also flattering to my skin tones.

I wear bright earth colors + C. I'm not sure. I wear bright earth colors as long.

8. For a purse, I usually carry:
  (A.) One good all-purpose bag that goes with all my clothes.
  B. Something fun and inexpensive that holds all the junk I carry around.
  C. Whatever matches my clothes.

9. The hair appliances I rely on include:
  A. A round brush and blow-dryer.
  (B.) I have all kinds of stuff, but I never use it.
  C. Electric rollers, hot combs, curling irons, crimper, dryers, and brushes.

I only comb my hair, I have a dryer for emergencies, as opposed to going somewhere where with my hair dripping wet. But I've been known to do that too.

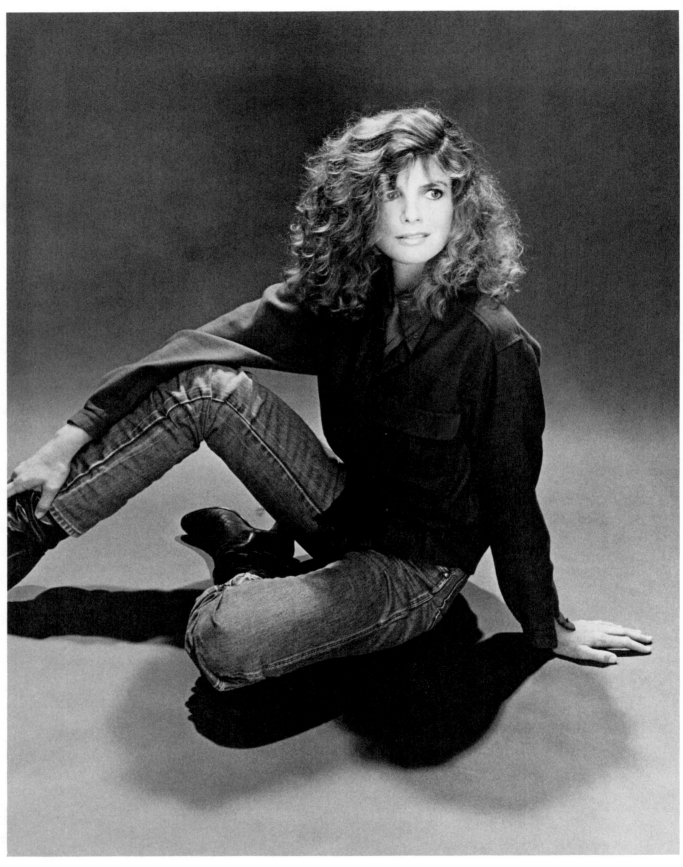

10. For breakfast, I:
    A. Grab something on the way to work or eat at my desk.
    B. Have cold cereal and fruit.
    C. Eat a light meal if I'm dieting or a little more if I'm having a late lunch.

none of these. I have hot lemon juice and water every once in a while an egg.

11. When I bathe, I:
    A. Take a shower first thing in the morning.
    (B.) Take a shower several times a day, after tennis or swimming.
    C. Take a leisurely bath.

12. I have help in my home:
    (A.) Never.
    B. Once or twice a week.
    C. Full time.

13. I put myself together:
    (A.) To please myself.
    B. To suit my life-style.
    C. To please my man.

It's primarily A but it's also C.

14. I work:
    A. Nine to five at a regular job.
    B. You think taking care of the kids isn't full-time work?
    C. Flexible hours or not at all.

15. My fingernails:
    (A.) Are manicured by me.
    B. Are kept short and neat for simplicity.
    C. I have done weekly.

16. When it comes to athletics:
    A. Weekends are the only time I have for recreational sports.
    (B.) I'd only be more active if I were training for the Olympics.
    C. I don't sweat.

17. If I have a little extra money to splurge with, I:
    (A.) Buy something I need.
    B. Get something for the kids.
    C. Buy something wonderful I've been dying to have.

18. My idea of the perfect vacation would be to:
    A. Travel to the major cities of Europe.
    (B.) Go hiking and backpacking.
    C. Escape to a spa.

A and B both appeal to me.

19. My bedtime is:
    A. After the 11:00 P.M. news.
    (B.) Early, after an exhausting day.
    C. Whenever the party's over.

Maybe A, but probably it's B

20. If I could sum up my beauty routine simply, I would say it's:
    (A.) Sensible.
    B. Practical.
    C. Time-consuming.

Jose says:
I'm very happy Katharine allowed me to cut her hair. She had one look that was very famous, but it was time to have something more than just plain long hair. Now she has a blunt cut, but the last two inches are slightly layered so the hair lies just the right way. She has a permanent, and for special occasions we curl her hair with tissue papers. I love her forehead and didn't want to give her bangs, so we part her hair on the side. This gives a fullness on top without resorting to bangs. And you can see her forehead. She has a unique look now, like an old-time movie star.

Pat Van Patten

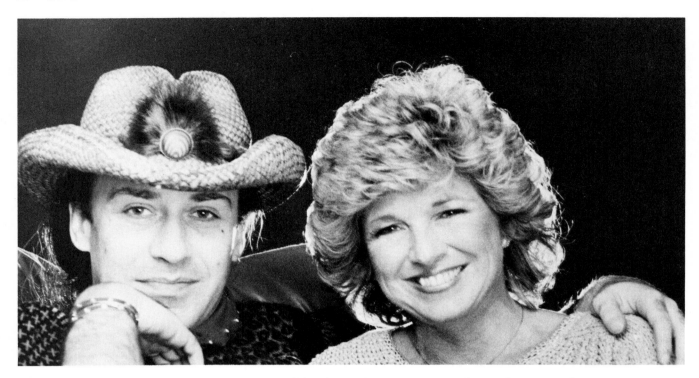

Pat Van Patten is a close friend of Farrah's; they play tennis together a lot. Farrah sent Pat to see me. She had very short hair when she came in, and I knew she kept it that way because of her active life-style, but really wanted longer hair so she could do more with it. I just had the feeling that she would be happier with more hair, and she said it was true, but her other hairstylists had always told her she couldn't wear longer hair because of her face shape.

Now Pat's hair is a little longer and it fits her busy life-style—she is still active in sports (she comes from a very "tennis" family!), she has a television show on cable TV, and she is the wife of actor Dick Van Patten. Her hair is layered and goes up and back, away from the face, for a very soft look. This keeps the hair out of her eyes when she plays tennis, which is very important for active women, but still gives her enough hair so she can use electric rollers if she wants to dress up her look.

It was Farrah's idea that Pat should stop coloring her hair. Now Aroxy just "tips" it, as Pat calls it. It's much younger-looking and is in keeping with the sun-drenched, California sporty look that's Pat's trademark.

JOSE EBER'S LIFE-STYLE QUIZ

Pat Van Patten

1. When I wake up in the morning:
  A. I look at the alarm clock and panic. I'm already late.
  (B.) Who needs an alarm clock? I'm up with the birds, or the kids, and ready to go.

I like to get up early; I like an early start because I don't always manage it.

I roll over and go back to sleep for another half hour because last night I was up too late

2. My regular morning routine:
  A. Takes no more than half an hour because I'm so busy.
  (B.) Is postponed until later in the day, because I'm out the door for tennis or carpool.
  C. Depends on what I'm doing during the day and what's cooking for the upcoming evening.

3. When I look in the mirror each morning I:
  A. Wish I had time to do something about what I see.
  B. Splash cold water on my face and check the condition of my skin.
  C. Study each line, blemish, and soft spot mercilessly, until I'm satisfied I know exactly how to best care for what I've seen.

D. I look in the mirror and plan to make an appointment with Jose.

4. First thing in the morning, my hair:
  A. Needs a wash and blow-dry.
  B. Kind of falls into place, because my haircut is easy to care for.
  C. Is almost perfect, because I just had it done yesterday.

Between A and B.

5. My hair:
  A. Gets cut whenever I'm in the mood or can't do a thing with it.
  (B.) Needs to be cut every four–six weeks; otherwise it's unmanageable.
  C. Is long to allow me to manage a variety of hairstyles depending on my needs so I just make sure the ends are trimmed frequently.

6. My hair color:
  A. Is something I've experimented with myself.
  B. Yuck! Ruin my hair with chemicals?
  (C.) Is done at the beauty shop every six weeks.

7. The colors I wear most frequently are:
  (A.) Neutrals that mix well in the business world: navy, burgundy, cream, and things that are "safe."
  B. Bright colors, I love 'em.
  C. Whatever the fashion mavens say is "in," as long as it's also flattering to my skin tones.

I love mauves, pinks and classics

8. For a purse, I usually carry:
  (A.) One good all-purpose bag that goes with all my clothes.
  B. Something fun and inexpensive that holds all the junk I carry around.
  C. Whatever matches my clothes.

9. The hair appliances I rely on include:
  A. A round brush and blow-dryer.
  B. I have all kinds of stuff, but I never use it.
  (C.) Electric rollers, hairpins, combs, clips, curling iron, crimper, dryers, and brushes.

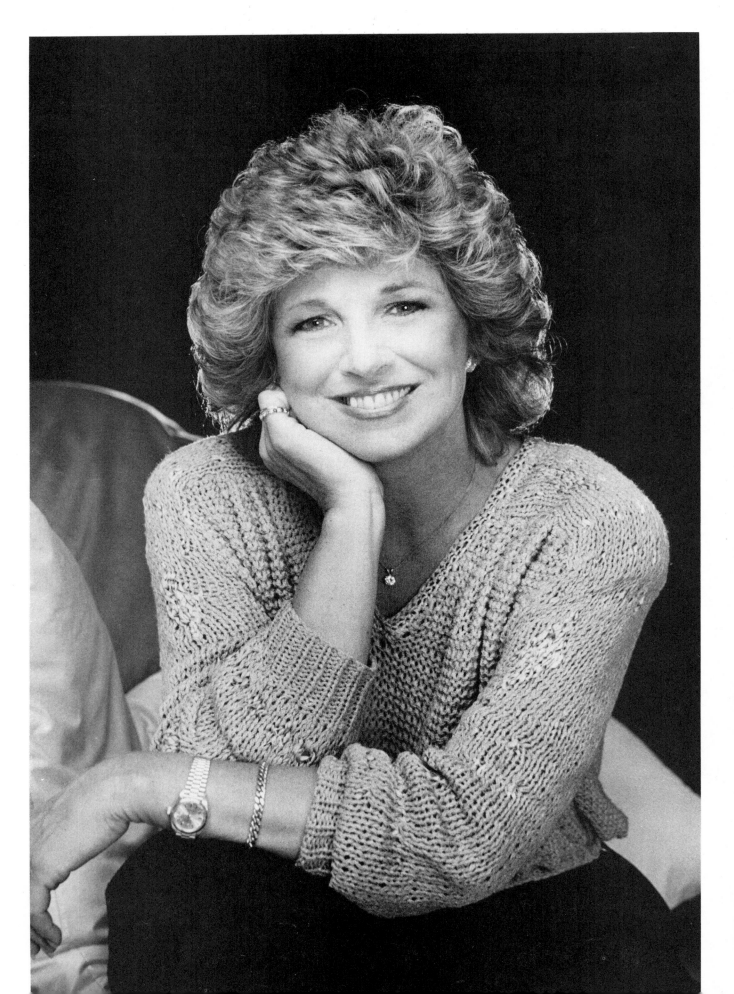

10. **For breakfast, I:**
    A. Grab something on the way to work or eat at my desk
    B. Have cold cereal and fruit.
    C. Eat a light meal if I'm dieting or a little more if I'm having a late lunch. *(C circled)*

11. **When I bathe, I:**
    A. Take a shower first thing in the morning.
    B. Take a shower several times a day, after tennis or swimming. *(B circled)*
    C. Take a leisurely bath.

    B and C; I shower a lot, and sauna and swim. *(handwritten)*

12. **I have help in my home:**
    A. Never.
    B. Once or twice a week. *(B circled)*
    C. Full time.

13. **I put myself together:**
    A. To please myself. *(A circled)*
    B. To suit my life-style.
    C. To please my man.

14. **I work:**
    A. Nine to five at a regular job.
    B. You think taking care of the kids isn't full time work?
    C. Flexible hours or not at all. *(struck through with handwritten line)*

15. **My fingernails:**
    A. Are manicured by me.

(handwritten at top of right column) B. I keep them short and neat for simplicity. C. I have done them self and have them done once in a while.

16. **When it comes to athletics:**
    A. Weekends are the only time I have for recreational sports.
    B. I'd only be more active if I were training for the Olympics. *(B circled)*
    C. I don't sweat.

17. **If I have a little extra money to splurge with, I:**
    A. Buy something I need. *(A circled)*
    B. Get something for the kids.
    C. Buy something wonderful I've been dying to have.

18. **My idea of the perfect vacation would be to:**
    A. Travel to the major cities of Europe. *(A circled)*
    B. Go hiking and backpacking.
    C. Escape to a spa.

19. **My bedtime is:**
    A. After the 11:00 P.M. news. *(A circled)*
    B. Early, after an exhausting day.
    C. Whenever the party's over.

20. **If I could sum up my beauty routine simply, I would say it's:**
    A. Sensible.
    B. Practical. *(B circled)*
    C. Time-consuming.

Jose says:
Patty's hair is cut to frame her face and give her a young look. She has a light permanent, and the hair is brushed away from her face in a way that is sporty but still feminine. The sides are pretty short, and all she has to do is blow-dry the hair away from her face and make sure she has a little fullness on top. The permanent helps there, because her hair is naturally very straight.

Stacey Winkler

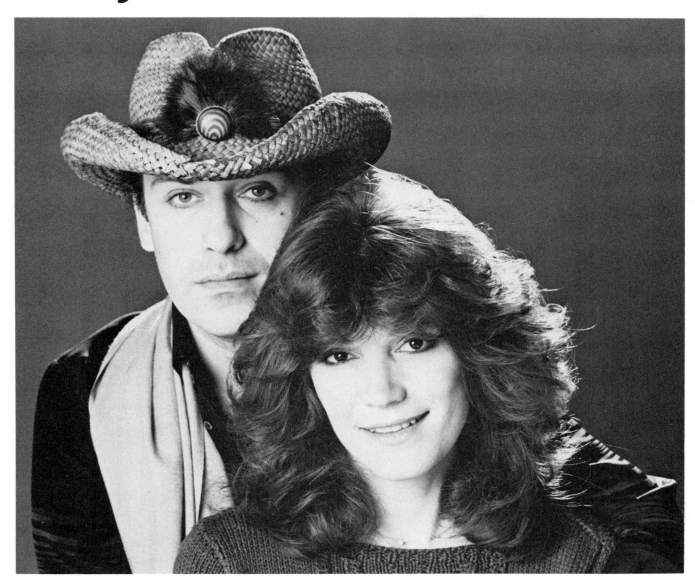

Stacey Winkler is to me the All-American woman and is one of my most representative clients. She is every woman. She does not go to work in an office—she gave up her own public-relations business a few years ago—but her day is crammed with work. She has two children, she is very busy helping her husband, who is the actor Henry Winkler, and she is very involved in many charities. As a result, her day is a nonstop combination of many different jobs. She wears every hat—like all wives.

Because she is so busy, Stacey is clearly a Life-style Red; she has no time for her hair. We keep her hair on the longish side, and even though it's trimmed regularly, I respect the fact that she likes it long and doesn't want to change it much. Her husband likes her to wear her hair in bunches, but I think it is sexy and practical down, with bangs. She has a full head of very thick hair, so she needs little maintenance with this cut.

After she washes her hair, she dries it with her hands, a blow-dryer, and a vent brush. She can turn her head upside down, blow and brush, and run out the door. In her case, the cut really matters, because it is the cut's responsibility to hold the hairstyle—as it is with that of all Life-style Reds. But she has her hair cut every six to eight weeks and has total freedom. And that, I think, is what everyone wants.

JOSE EBER'S LIFE-STYLE QUIZ

Stacy Winkler

1. **When I wake up in the morning:**
   A. I look at the alarm clock and panic. I'm already late.
   B. Who needs an alarm clock? I'm up with the birds, or the kids, and ready to go.
   C. I roll over and go back to sleep for another half hour because last night really was a bit too much.

2. **My regular morning routine:**
   A. Takes no more than half an hour because I'm so busy.
   B. Is postponed until later in the day, because I'm out the door for tennis or carpool.
   C. Depends on what I'm doing during the day and what's cooking for the upcoming evening.

3. **When I look in the mirror each morning I:**
   A. Wish I had time to do something about what I see.
   B. Splash cold water on my face and check the condition of my skin.
   C. Study each line, blemish, and soft spot mercilessly, until I'm satisfied I know exactly how to best care for what I've seen.

4. **First thing in the morning, my hair:**
   A. Needs a wash and blow-dry.
   B. Kind of falls into place, because my haircut is easy to care for.
   C. Is almost perfect, because I just had it done yesterday.

5. **My hair:**
   A. Gets cut whenever I'm in the mood or can't do a thing with it.
   B. Needs to be cut every four–six weeks; otherwise it's unmanageable.
   C. Is long to allow me to manage a variety of hairstyles depending on my needs so I just make sure the ends are trimmed frequently.

6. **My hair color:**
   A. Is something I've experimented with myself.
   B. Yuck! Ruin my hair with chemicals?
   C. Is done at the beauty shop every six weeks. *my hair color is natural.*

7. **The colors I wear most frequently are:**
   A. Neutrals that mix well in the business world: navy, burgundy, cream, and things that are "safe."
   B. Bright colors, I love 'em.
   C. Whatever the fashion mavens say is "in," as long as it's also flattering to my skin tones.

8. **For a purse, I usually carry:**
   A. One good all purpose bag that goes with all my clothes.
   B. Something fun and inexpensive that's holds all the stuff I carry around.
   C. Whatever matches my clothes.

   I like color but it depends on whether I have time to change bags.

9. **The hair appliances I rely on include:**
   A. A round brush and blow-dryer.
   B. I have all kinds of stuff, but I never use it.
   C. Electric rollers, hairpins, combs, clips, curling iron, crimper, dryers, and brushes.

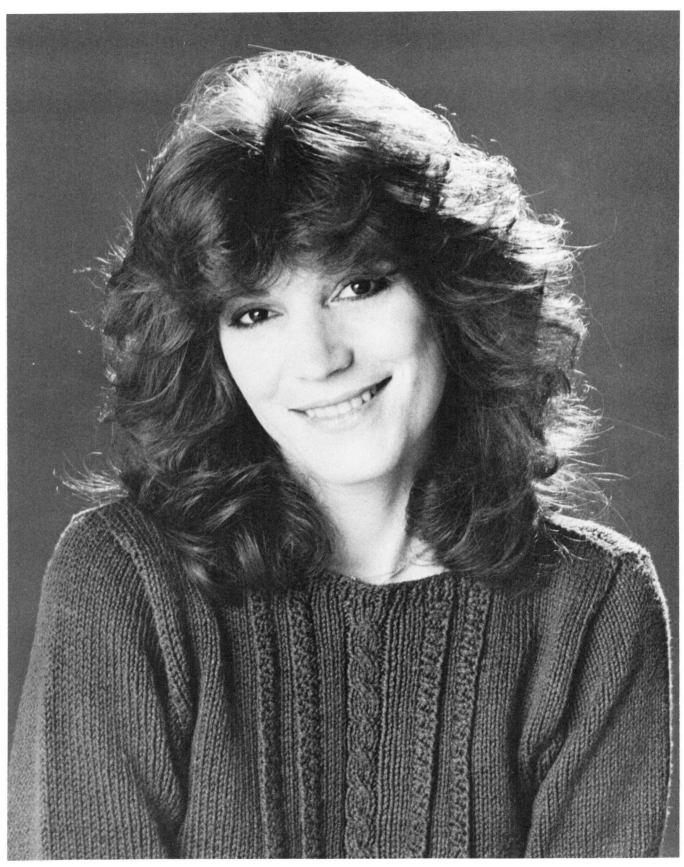

10. **For breakfast, I:**
    A. Grab something on the way to work or eat at my desk.
    B. Have cold cereal and fruit.
    C. Eat a light meal if I'm dieting or a little more if I'm having a late lunch.

    I eat nothing for breakfast. I have a cup of tea.

11. **When I bathe, I:**
    A. Take a shower first thing in the morning.
    B. Have a shower set at all times in the morning or nighttime.
    C. Take a leisurely bath.

    It depends on how cramped I am, and other things like that. I shower when I have things to do and I like something late in the afternoon if I get to take a bath late in the afternoon. I have time.

12. **I have help in my home:**
    A. Never.
    B. Once or twice a week.
    (C.) Full time.

13. **I put myself together:**
    (A.) To please myself.
    B. To suit my life-style.
    C. To please my man.

    It's a combination of all three

14. **I work:**
    A. Nine to five at a regular job.
    B. Part-time, taking care of the kids.
    C. Full-time at work.
    D. Flexible hours or not at all.

    I do a lot of things, so I'm really in all three of these categories. I don't go out to work at an office, but my day is full with children and various projects and helping my husband.

15. **My fingernails:**
    A. Are manicured by me.

    B. Are kept short and neat for simplicity.
    (C.) I have done weekly.

16. **When it comes to athletics:**
    A. Weekends are the only time I have for recreational sports.
    B. I'd only be more active if I were training for the Olympics.
    C. I don't sweat.

    I have a bad back.

17. **If I have a little extra money to splurge with, I:**
    A. Buy something I need.
    (B.) Get something for the kids.
    C. Buy something wonderful I've been dying to have.

18. **My idea of the perfect vacation would be to:**
    A. Travel to the major cities of Europe.
    B. Go hiking or backpacking.
    C. Go away to a spa.
    D. *go someplace with my husband where no phones are ringing it's quiet and*

19. **My bedtime is:**
    A. After the 11:00 P.M. news.
    B. Early, after an exhausting day.
    C. Whenever the party's over.
    D. *Between 12:30 and 1:00 A.M.*

20. **If I could sum up my beauty routine simply, I would say it's:**
    A. Sensible.
    (B.) Practical.
    C. Time-consuming.

Jose says:

Stacey has incredibly beautiful long red hair which I try to keep very simple for her, because she has no time. She has children and a famous husband and is always doing so much, you can't believe it. The long hair makes her feel more feminine and sexy, and its weight keeps the curl down, so it doesn't look curly. This length is easier to care for than short hair, and Stacey is done in less than ten minutes. She just brushes her hair upside down, shakes her head, and that's it. I cut wide bangs to emphasize her cheekbones and to make sure her face isn't covered by her hair. The bangs are also wide enough to give her a little fullness on the top of her head.

Life-style Green

PROFILE

The difference between a Life-style Green and a Life-style Red woman sometimes appears to be very subtle, and many women who take my Life-style Quiz claim to fall someplace between the two categories. So let me make it easier for you right now.

The Life-style Green woman almost invariably leaves the house to go to a job. She's gone all day, does not change her clothes, and doesn't return home until the evening. If she uses her lunch hour for a game of racquetball, she's Life-style Red. If she spends her lunch hour at a business meeting, doing errands, or getting extra work done, she's a Life-style Green. Life-style Greens only have time for sports on the weekends.

What else can I tell you about the Green woman?

Well, let me see, darling.

The Green woman is more in control of her morning, her beauty routine, and her life than the Red woman. The Red woman is a victim of circumstance and outside influences (and often children); the Green woman may have children, but she usually has help with them. She makes time for her "look" and takes a lot of care, to be sure that when she leaves the house it will last all day. Her clothes are often chosen for the business world and may be a bit on the safe side if her job demands that. Weekends and evenings she dresses for herself, but during the day she is wearing her dress-for-success suit or the kind of clothes her peers expect. Each job has its own type of uniform, and the Green woman is very conscious of what she should be wearing to work and how she wants to present herself to the public.

The Green woman has between thirty and sixty minutes for her total morning routine, but only because her time is limited. She must get to work on time! Her hair does not need to be a certain length hair or cut in a cookie-cutter style. For the Green woman, when she chooses the hairstyle that goes with the variables appropriate for her, the most important thing is that the hair be well cut. Greens are not looking for wash-and-wear hair (life Life-style Reds); they are looking for staying power.

You need to look pretty all day, with a cut that is sophisticated and versatile enough to go from day to night. The cut should look right at a meeting, at a lunch, and still be holding up after you've stopped by the market and gotten home to cook dinner or prepare for your date. You don't want to look like a wilted flower for your husband or boyfriend, darling.

The cut has to be good enough to last and to allow you to dress it up or down, depending on your need. The cut shouldn't be too sporty; it must be appealing and sexy without being inappropriate for a business setting. It should please men and women, and you most of all.

The Green woman is often expecting magic and doesn't realize that she has to take time to create her own. She cannot snap her fingers and look good all day, but if she takes a little time, she will be quite pleased with her lasting look. Life-Style Greens tend to wander from one hairstyle to another and then wish they still had their old one, because it was better or easier to care for, even though they were bored with it and wanted the change. They don't regulate their beauty appointments but let their look have a life of its own, which is part of their charm. They're also very big on taking their beauty rituals into their own hands—Life-style Greens are the ones who like to do their own hair color at home (or have a friend come over to do it), give themselves a permanent, and even cut their own hair. Usually they do these things because they think that the products on the market now are so easy to use that they can manage them, and they will save some money and time. Since they have such erratic beauty-parlor habits, when they suddenly decide it's time for a haircut or they need a change, they want it immediately—even if it's one o'clock in the morning! Because they are so competent in the business world, they think they can do anything. It is usually Life-style Greens who come to me in a panic or in tears, asking me to fix whatever thay have botched up. Life-style Greens are also the ones who come to me, like what they get, and then think their hair will never grow, and they don't have to come back for six months. Then they wonder why they don't look the same in three months and can't do anything with their hair.

But don't get me wrong—Life-style Greens are vibrant and exciting people, and I do love them. They usually walk in carrying a very good handbag, the expensive kind, or even a designer bag. It may be years old and well worn, but it still looks good. Sometimes they bring a calendar or work schedule or computer printout or some other kind of work, because they're so busy, they are always doing two things at once.

Greens are the kind of people who eat on the run and often don't have a good meal. They're not usually dieting (like Blues), but they don't give themselves enough time to eat properly, so they often grab a bite or have candy bars and junk food—all of which is terrible for the skin, the hair, and your overall beauty.

Women in this life-style category almost always work and are very careful with their money. If they have a little extra, they usually spend it carefully and wisely, on something they need, rather than on a silly luxury. They believe in savings accounts or rainy-day funds and would rarely blow a week's salary on anything.

Even during their time off, Greens don't relax much. They choose a vacation that's as busy as their life-style, and hate to relax or go on trips where they do nothing. Even window-shopping is fun for them—it's better than doing nothing. Sports are for weekends. They're more likely to prefer one-on-one sports than group sports—they'll take jogging over being a member of the company softball team.

They don't like to waste time and have little patience with people who do, and they like to do things their own way. Greens are usually self-starters, who don't need to be told to get going on a project. They're bright and creative and usually come up with the best ideas for entertainment. But they're independent also, and would never go along with a group just to be one of the gang. Yet, because they work, they have respect for authority and are usually careful to fit comfortably into the group.

HOW TO SHAMPOO YOUR HAIR

Most Greens wash their hair every morning, although sometimes, if their hair is not too greasy, they will do it every other morning. I even know Greens who wash their hair one day and condition it the next, so they rotate their hair treatments.

Life-style Greens are tempted to take shortcuts in the shampoo department, but they really have to be careful that their hair is washed as often as it needs to be. They may leave the house looking fine and end up feeling very embarrassed late in the afternoon. It's better to take the time to shampoo daily, with a mild shampoo. Then you always look perfect and won't have to worry about your hair later in the day—because we all know that Green women will have no time then to fix their hair!

Have several mild shampoos on hand, so you can alternate them. One shampooing is plenty; you do not need two, because you wash your hair every day. Use lots of water when you rinse it. The shower is the best place for a Green to shampoo. Reds may be tempted to shampoo in the sink, but Greens will naturally gravitate toward the shower first thing in the morning.

Virgin hair will need very little extra care. A light conditioner (creme rinse) can be used every day or every other day, depending on need. Too much creme rinse will make the hair too soft, and then it will not have the body to last all day long and stay properly styled. (Body is one reason many Greens like to shampoo every other day—when their hair is a little bit dirty, it holds its shape better. This is a personal decision.)

Creme rinse should go mostly on the ends and in the damaged areas, because the hair's body will come from the roots, and you don't want to destroy the body or the shape-holding capacity of your haircut.

If your hair is so dry or damaged that creme rinse does not help and is making your hair too soft, stop this treatment immediately. Skip the regular creme rinses and save your time and money. Instead, give yourself deep-conditioning treatments (and check your diet and weather variables) to improve the general condition of your hair without destroying its ability to stand up to your busy day.

Greens very much like to be in charge of their own beauty routines, and a deep conditioning is one treatment you can't mess up yourself. You can save the time and money you'd spend at a salon for this treatment. You may want to purchase a deep conditioner from your hairdresser, at your local drugstore, or use a homemade variety such as mayonnaise or mineral oil or Crisco. Whatever you use, give yourself a deep conditioning for at least twenty minutes, and preferably thirty, once a week.

If you are a Life-style Green with no children or social obligations, you may want to have a deep-conditioning treatment followed by a shampoo, in the evening. Towel-dry your hair, and in the morning you can wet it in the shower or with a spritzer bottle, and use your shower time to try electric rollers or something special. (Or you can use your shower time to sleep ten minutes longer.)

CONDITIONING

Conditioning is very important to your hair, because your hair needs to stay in place and it also needs to look good. It's very hard to work in the business world and not be judged by your appearance. And damaged hair does not impress anyone.

The problem with Life-style Greens and conditioning is that, while they set aside an hour in the morning to get dressed and complete their beauty look, they rarely give themselves any other time for beauty. They tend to neglect something as important as conditioning until it's too late.

If your hair is bleached or permed, you will definitely have to condition it well and often, so maybe you should rethink your schedule a little bit. Your family or your boyfriend will have to get used to your taking a little extra time to walk around the house with your hair in aluminum foil and a scarf. Let them tease you! As long as you condition your hair, it doesn't matter how much they joke.

HOW TO DRY YOUR HAIR

The blow-dryer is the Green Woman's most often-used tool for drying her hair. She was thrilled to be liberated from old-fashioned hood hair dryers, because blow-drying is usually quicker and easier for her and has been a boon in advancing her out of the Life-style Blue category, where she didn't have the time to be.

I do not recommend wash-and-wear hair for Life-style Greens, although it is an option. Should they choose this beauty look, they will of course not need to worry about drying their hair. But I like the Green woman to look "done" in a casual way, and this means a thorough and careful drying with a blow-dryer and a brush, so that shape and style can be put into the hair by the heat of the dryer and the shape of the brush.

Greens should get a lesson on drying from their stylist each time they get a new hairstyle, but generally they should dry the hair framing the face first. This will set up the shape of the hairstyle, and if they aren't as thorough with the crown or back, they may be able to survive and still look fine. It's unlikely that a Life-style Green will be using hot rollers, but she may need a curling iron, once her hair is shaped with the blow-dryer.

If you have short hair all over or on top, you may want to let your hair dry naturally while you put on your makeup, and then touch up the ends with your trusty curling iron.

PERMANENTS

Staying power is the most important element in a Life-style Green's hairstyle, so a light perm or body wave may be what you need, especially if your hair is thin or fine. You may just want to have the permanent solution applied to the roots, so you can have a straight hairstyle that will have a little more strength to it. This will add to its staying power.

I do not recommend that the Life-style Green woman give herself a home permanent, even though she will be tempted. She could leave the solution on too long or perm more areas than necessary. What she must do is get her calendar organized enough so she can take some time off from work or family—a weekend, if need be—or find a salon that is open all night, to have the job done professionally.

COLORING

I strongly recommend coloring for Life-style Greens, because it will probably give your hair more body, which will give it more staying power. And coloring can be done at home to the satisfaction of every Green woman. Highlighting adds extra body and doesn't bog you down with a commitment to having to constantly color your roots. Henna is good here, even if it's the kind with no additional color. It adds body.

Just remember that you are out in public and your image is extremely important. You don't want any dark new growth sneaking up under your dress-for-success hairstyle. And be sure to deep-condition your colored hair.

TO SPRAY OR NOT TO SPRAY

I cannot stress to you how much I don't like hair spray, and I do not recommend that anyone use it. It dries and damages the hair, and when used too often it can create terrible problems. Besides, I think the stiff look is passé and should be forgotten. But I do have a hair-spray trick that is perfect for Life-style Greens. Like any trick, this is good once in a while, not all the time. If you do it too often, you will have damaged hair and be very miserable. Now on to the trick.

Fluff or tease up your hair and bend over. Shake your hair and then spray it lightly—with the hair spray held out as far as you can reach—from underneath. Then shake your hair with your fingers and stand upright. Now comb it. This will give your hair some extra staying power if you need it to last into the night.

SUPPLIES

Daily
soft shampoo (several varieties, to alternate)
blow-dryer

Often
creme rinse
deep conditioner
aluminum foil
curling iron

Occasionally
electric rollers
tissue paper or tissues for curling process

Disaster days
hats
combs

YOUR MORNING SCHEDULE

- 7:00–7:30 A.M. Wake up
- Immediately shower and wash hair (includes creme rinse or conditioning): 20 minutes
- Blow-dry and style hair: 20 minutes
- Makeup: 10 minutes
- Dress and get briefcase: 10 minutes

- Total beauty routine: 60 minutes
  OFF TO WORK

Sandra Dee

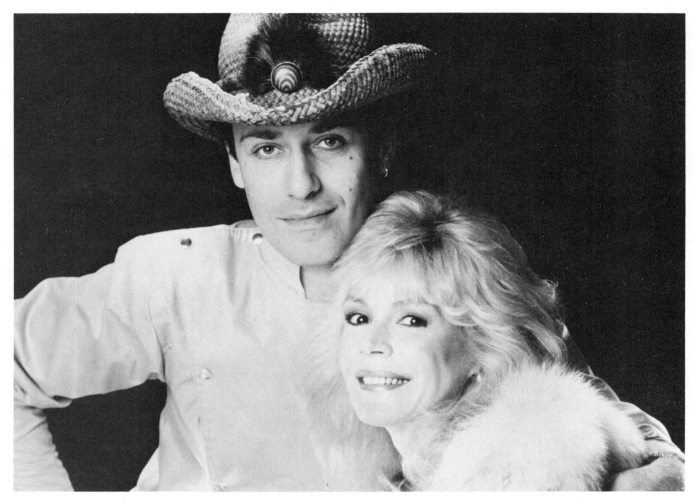

I first went to Jose when I was bald. My hair was broken into a million pieces, and I had to use combs to cover the spots where my head showed through. You have to remember that my hair has been taken care of by the studios since I was eleven years old. That's a lot of years of overbleaching and overtoning. Then I either bumped into Ali MacGraw at exercise class or read a magazine article about the trouble she had with her hair and I found out about Jose.

I simply said to him, "Help." I wanted him just to do whatever he had to so I could hold my hair together. I knew I was going to have to go to a short haircut, which I don't like, but we had to save my hair.

Three weeks after Jose first cut it, I started to go to his colorist Araxy, who straightened out the color and the condition. What used to take two hours in terms of color now takes twenty minutes. I also get henna for conditioning, and Araxy's special brew I don't like creme rinses, because they leave my hair limp, but I do condition at home after I shampoo, and I switch brands to make them work better.

Letting Jose cut my hair off was the best thing I ever did. Now my hair is thicker than I ever would have thought possible. When my hair is wet, I can squeeze it in place and look great, because of the way it's cut. Most of us in the business go to Jose for that fantastic cut. I don't like hair that looks done.

I treat my hair better than I treat any other part of my body, because now I know how fragile it is. You've got to treat your hair like breakable porcelain, because it will break. I was on the road for seven months and sometimes had my hair done three or four times a day. That's what finally did my hair in. Now I don't let anyone lift a scissors to me, even if it's to cut a string, unless it's Jose.

JOSE EBER'S LIFE-STYLE QUIZ

Sandra Dee

1. **When I wake up in the morning:**
   A. I look at the alarm clock and panic. I'm already late.
   B. (circled) Who needs an alarm clock? I'm up with the birds, or the kids, and ready to go.

   that roll over and go back to sleep for another half hour because last night... it without a doubt — cruise before the service call me. I'm up... really was a bit too much.

2. **My regular morning routine:**
   A. Takes no more than half an hour because I'm so busy.
   B. Is postponed until later in the day, because I'm out the door for tennis or carpool.
   C. (circled) Depends on what I'm doing during the day and what's cooking for the upcoming evening.

3. **When I look in the mirror each morning I:**
   A. Wish I had time to do something about what I see.
   B. Splash cold water on my face and check the condition of my skin.
   C. (circled) Study each line, blemish, and soft spot mercilessly, until I'm satisfied I know exactly how to best care for what I've seen.

   Well, I don't scrutinize, but I look.

4. **First thing in the morning, my hair:**
   A. (circled) Needs a wash and blow-dry.
   B. Kind of falls into place because my haircut is easy to care for.
   C. Is almost perfect because I just wash it down every day.

   I have fine and oily scalp and even though it's a paradox it means dry hair and I have to wash my hair every single stinking day.

5. **My hair:**
   A. Gets cut whenever I'm in the mood or can't do a thing with it.
   B. (circled) Needs to be cut every four–six weeks; otherwise it's unmanageable.
   C. Is long to allow me to manage a variety of hairstyles depending on my needs so I just make sure the ends are trimmed frequently.

6. **My hair color:**
   A. Is something I've experimented with myself.
   B. Yuck! Ruin my hair with chemicals?
   C. Is done at the beauty shop every six weeks.

   B and C. My hair has been ruined by chemicals, but now Aroxy does my color at Jose's and everything is under control.

7. **The colors I wear most frequently are:**
   A. Neutrals that mix well in the business world: navy, burgundy, cream, and things that are "safe."
   B. (circled) Bright colors, I love 'em.
   C. Whatever the fashion mavens say is "in" as long as it's also flattering to my skin tones.

   I love colors and wear most of them.

8. **For a purse, I usually carry:**
   A. One good all-purpose bag that goes with all my clothes.
   B. Something fun and inexpensive that holds all the junk I carry around.
   C. Whatever matches my clothes.

   All three.

9. **The hair appliances I rely on include:**
   A. A round brush and blow-dryer.
   B. (circled) I have all kinds of stuff, but I never use it.
   C. Electric rollers, hairpins, combs, clips, curling iron, crimper, dryers, and brushes.

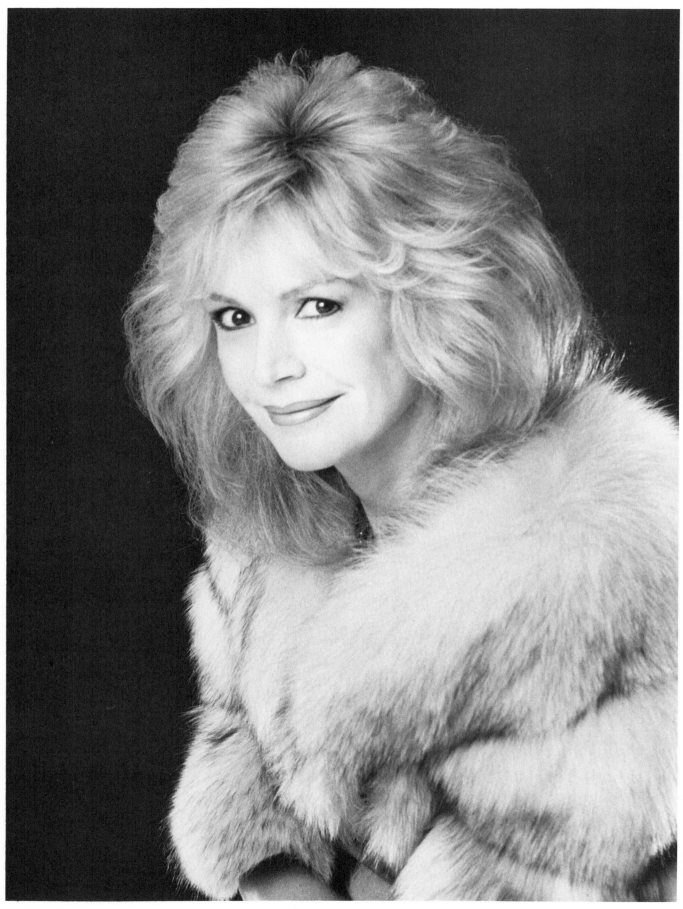

10. For breakfast, I:

A. Grab something on the way to work or eat at my desk.

B. Have cold cereal and fruit.

C. Eat a light meal if I'm dieting or a little more if I'm having a late lunch.

D. I eat nothing or maybe have some coffee in the morning.

11. When I bathe, I:

(A.) Take a shower first thing in the morning.

B. Take a shower several times a day, after tennis or swimming.

C. Take a leisurely bath.

12. I have help in my home:

A. Never.

B. Once or twice a week.

(C.) Full time.

13. I put myself together:

(A.) To please myself.

B. To suit my life-style.

C. To please my man.

14. I work:

A. Nine to five at a regular job.

B. You think taking care of the kids isn't full-time work?

C. Flexible hours or not at all.

15. My fingernails:

A. Are manicured by me.

B. Are kept short and neat for simplicity. *they're my own and I get them done regularly*

(C.) I have done weekly.

16. When it comes to athletics:

A. Weekends are the only time I have for recreational sports.

(B.) I'd only be more active if I were training for the Olympics.

C. I don't sweat.

17. If I have a little extra money to splurge with, I:

A. Buy something I need.

(B.) Get something for the kids.

C. Buy something wonderful I've been dying to have.

B and C

18. My idea of the perfect vacation would be to:

A. Travel to the major cities of Europe.

B. Go hiking and backpacking.

C. Escape to a spa.

D. Stay at home. How about D. I've been all over the world and seen everything. It's these kids, because I was working all the time. I have everything I need at home.

19. My bedtime is:

A. After the 11:00 P.M. news.

(B.) Early, after an exhausting day.

C. Whenever the party's over.

20. If I could sum up my beauty routine simply, I would say it's:

(A.) Sensible.

B. Practical.

C. Time-consuming.

Jose Eber says:

We layer Sandra's hair all the way. Her face is so petite that she needs volume all over the place but still has to have a hairstyle that is easy to care for and versatile. This haircut can dry naturally; then Sandra uses electric rollers and brushes out her hair, away from the face. She gets the fullness she needs and still has length, so she can do lots of things with her hair.

Chana Eber

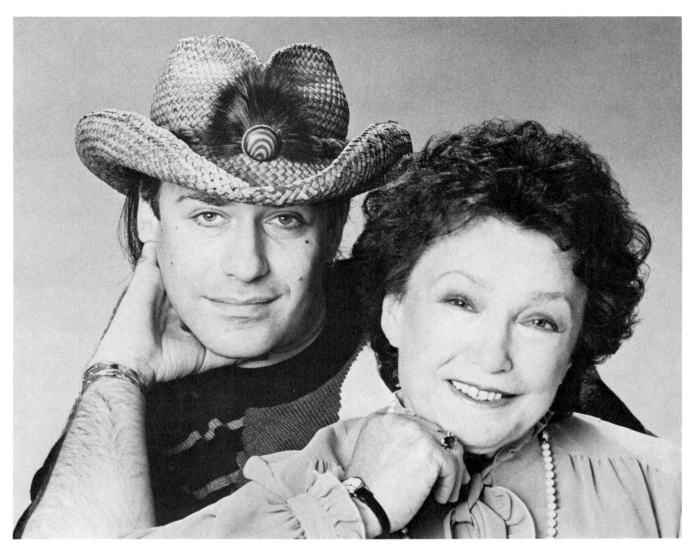

Chana Eber is my mother, and she lives part of the year in Europe, part of the year in Los Angeles, and part of the year in Israel, where my sister, Esther, lives. I have been doing her hair since I was thirteen. We used to sit in front of the television set while the other kids were outside playing, and I would style my mother's hair like the stars' we saw on television. My mother was very good with her own hair—she still is—but I liked to do it, and she let me, because she saw that I knew what I was doing.

When I went to camp, it was the same thing. I always did all the girls' hair.

Now Mama's beauty routine is very simple. She doesn't have much time for her hair and makeup and she is very European in her routine. She uses regular not electric rollers, and washes her hair every other day or every third day. In between washings, if she is going out, she'll put in a few rollers for ten or fifteen minutes. She does her hair herself, unless it's some special occasion, then I will do it. The color is done at the shop.

JOSE EBER'S LIFE-STYLE QUIZ   *Chana Eber*

1. **When I wake up in the morning:**
   A. I look at the alarm clock and panic. I'm already late.
   B. (circled) Who needs an alarm clock? I'm up with the birds, or the kids, and ready to go.
   C. I roll over and go back to sleep for another half hour because last night really was a bit too much.

2. **My regular morning routine:**
   A. (circled) Takes no more than half an hour because I'm so busy.
   B. Is postponed until later in the day, because I'm out the door for tennis or carpool.
   C. Depends on what I'm doing during the day and what's cooking for the upcoming evening.

3. **When I look in the mirror each morning I:**
   A. Wish I had time to do something about what I see.
   B. (circled) Splash cold water on my face and check the condition of my skin.
   C. Study each line, blemish, and soft spot mercilessly, until I'm satisfied I know exactly how to best care for what I've seen.

4. **First thing in the morning, my hair:**
   A. Needs a wash and blow-dry.
   B. (circled) Kind of falls into place, because my haircut is easy to care for.
   C. Is almost perfect, because I just had it done yesterday.

5. **My hair:**
   A. Gets cut whenever I'm in the mood or can't do a thing with it.
   B. (circled) Needs to be cut every four–six weeks; otherwise it's unmanageable.
   C. Is long to allow me to manage a variety of hairstyles depending on my needs so I just make sure the ends are trimmed frequently.

6. **My hair color:**
   A. Is something I've experimented with myself.
   B. Yuck! Ruin my hair with chemicals?
   C. (circled) Is done at the beauty shop every six weeks.

7. **The colors I wear most frequently are:**
   A. (circled) Neutrals that mix well in the business world: navy, burgundy, cream, and things that are "safe."
   B. Bright colors, I love 'em.
   C. Whatever the fashion mavens say is "in," as long as it's also flattering to my skin tones.

8. **For a purse, I usually carry:**
   A. (circled) One good all-purpose bag that goes with all my clothes.
   B. Something fun and inexpensive that holds all the junk I carry around.
   C. Whatever matches my clothes.

9. **The hair appliances I rely on include:**
   A. A round brush and blow-dryer.
   B. I have all kinds of stuff, but I never use it.
   C. Electric rollers, hairpins, combs, clips, curling iron, crimper, dryers, and brushes.

Rouleaux.

SHAKE YOUR HEAD, DARLING

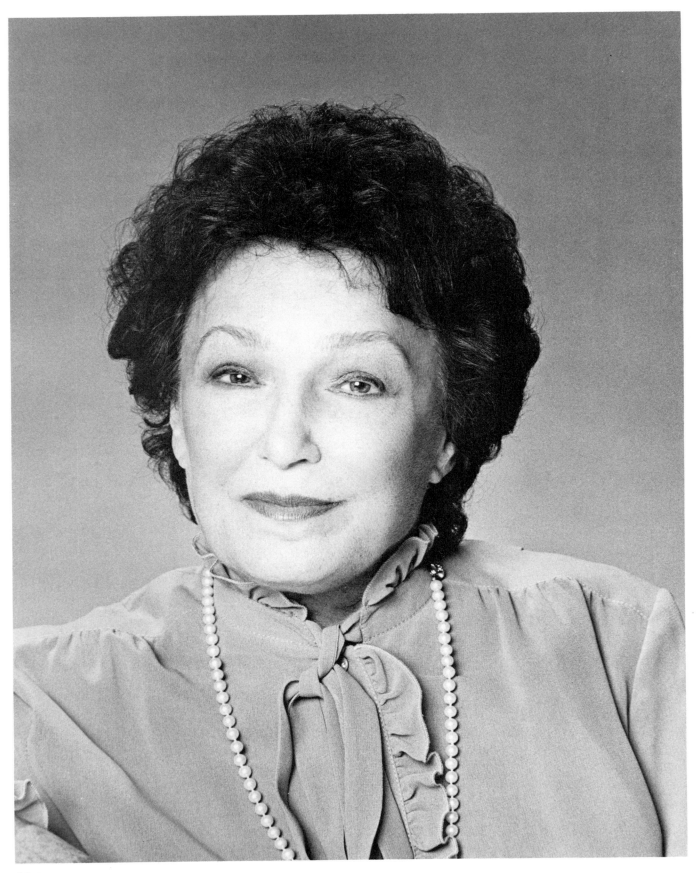

10. **For breakfast, I:**
    A. Grab something on the way to work or eat at my desk
    B. Have cold cereal and fruit.
    C. Eat a light meal if I'm dieting or a little more if I'm having a late lunch.

    Thé et toast.

11. **When I bathe, I:**
    (A.) Take a shower first thing in the morning.
    B. Take a shower several times a day, after tennis or swimming.
    C. Take a leisurely bath.

12. **I have help in my home:**
    A. Never.
    (B.) Once or twice a week.
    C. Full time.

13. **I put myself together:**
    A. To please myself.
    (B.) To suit my life-style.
    C. To please my man.

14. **I work:**
    A. Nine to five at a regular job.
    B. You think taking care of the kids isn't full-time work?
    (C.) Flexible hours or not at all.

    Je ne travaille pas.

15. **My fingernails:**
    A. Are manicured by me.

(B.) Are kept short and neat for simplicity.
    C. I have done weekly.

16. **When it comes to athletics:**
    A. Weekends are the only time I have for recreational sports.
    B. I'd only be more active if I were training for the Olympics.
    (C.) I don't sweat.

17. **If I have a little extra money to splurge with, I:**
    A. Buy something I need.
    (B.) Get something for the kids.
    C. Buy something wonderful I've been dying to have.

    Mon fils.

18. **My idea of the perfect vacation would be to:**
    A. Travel to the major cities of Europe.
    B. Go hiking and backpacking.
    C. Escape to a spa.

    D. Visiter mes enfants.

19. **My bedtime is:**
    (A.) After the 11:00 P.M. news.
    B. Early, after an exhausting day.
    C. Whenever the party's over.

20. **If I could sum up my beauty routine simply, I would say it's:**
    A. Sensible.
    (B.) Practical.
    C. Time-consuming.

Jose says:
Mama feels better in short hair, because it makes her life easier and she doesn't have to spend too much time on it. She has stick-straight hair, so she needs a light permanent. I don't pull the hair too far away from the face, because I think her hairline is too high, and I like to hide that. Also, her neck is short, so I don't like too much hair to hide it.

105

Lisa Hartman

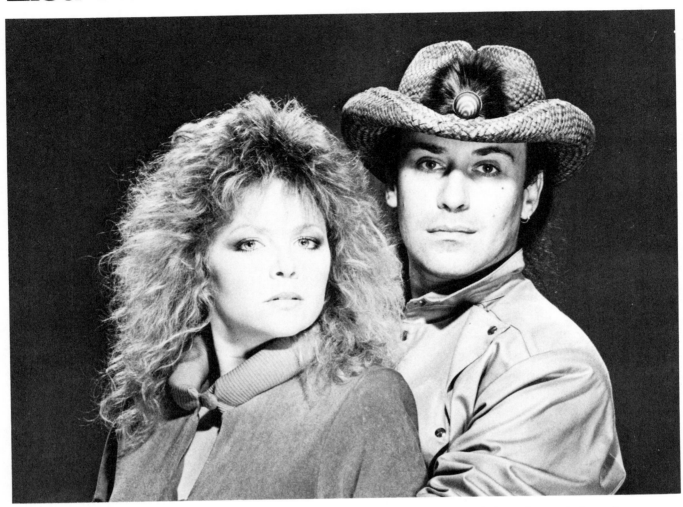

I met Jose through some mutal friends, and right away I began to ask him his opinion about my hair and what to do with it in terms of work. Sometimes I'm in movies and sometimes I perform live, and I always want the latest styles, but I want them to look good and be right for me. I don't want to look passé, but I don't want to look too extreme, either. The hairstyle has to be becoming, and that's what I rely on Jose for. He also makes me laugh.

He knows what looks best on me, he gives me good advice, and he's always able to combine the right hairstyle with my career and my activities. I'm busy running around all the time and I'm active athletically, so I need a hairstyle that isn't much bother. And Jose thinks of all these things and still makes me look good. That's what I call a real friend.

JOSE EBER'S LIFE-STYLE QUIZ   *Lisa Hartman*

1. **When I wake up in the morning:**
   A. I look at the alarm clock and panic. I'm already late.
   B. Who needs an alarm clock? I'm up with the birds, or the kids, and ready to go.
   C. *(circled)* I roll over and go back to sleep for another half hour because last night really was a bit too much.

2. **My regular morning routine:**
   A. Takes no more than half an hour because I'm so busy.
   B. Is postponed until later in the day, because I'm out the door for tennis or carpool.
   C. *(circled)* Depends on what I'm doing during the day and what's cooking for the upcoming evening.

3. **When I look in the mirror each morning I:**
   A. Wish I had time to do something about what I see.
   B. *(circled)* Splash cold water on my face and check the condition of my skin.
   C. Study each line, blemish, and soft spot mercilessly, until I'm satisfied I know exactly how to best care for what I've seen. *and drink orange juice.*

4. **First thing in the morning, my hair:**
   A. *(circled)* Needs a wash and blow-dry.
   B. Kind of falls into place, because my haircut is easy to care for.
   C. Is almost perfect, because I just had it done yesterday.
   No blow dry; it dries naturally.

5. **My hair:**
   A. *(circled)* Gets cut whenever I'm in the mood or can't do a thing with it.
   B. Needs to be cut every four-six weeks; otherwise it's unmanageable.
   C. Is long to allow me to manage a variety of hairstyles depending on my needs so I just make sure the ends are trimmed frequently.

6. **My hair color:**
   A. Is something I've experimented with myself.
   B. Yuck! Ruin my hair with chemicals?
   C. *(circled)* Is done at the beauty shop every six weeks. *whenever it needs it.*

7. **The colors I wear most frequently are:**
   A. Neutrals that mix well in the business world: navy, burgundy, cream, and things that are "safe."
   B. *(circled)* Bright colors, I love 'em.
   C. Whatever the fashion mavens say is "in," as long as it's also flattering to my skin tones.

8. **For a purse, I usually carry:**
   A. *(circled)* One good all-purpose bag that goes with all my clothes.
   B. Something fun and inexpensive that holds all the junk I carry around.
   C. Whatever matches my clothes.

9. **The hair appliances I rely on include:**
   A. *(circled)* A round brush and blow-dryer.
   B. I have all kinds of stuff, but I never use it.
   C. Electric rollers, hairpins, combs, clips, curling iron, crimper, dryers, and brushes.

107

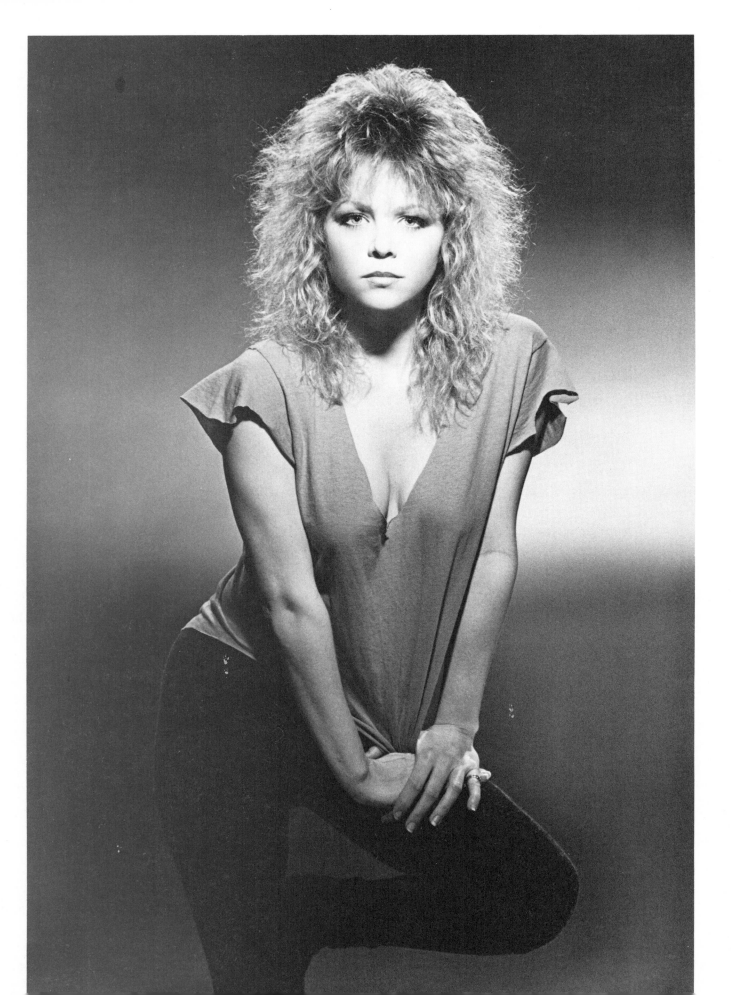

10. **For breakfast, I:**
    A. Grab something on the way to work or eat at my desk
    B. *(circled)* Have cold cereal and fruit.
    C. Eat a light meal if I'm dieting or a little more if I'm having a late lunch.
    D. Just orange juice and occasionally fruit.

11. **When I bathe, I:**
    A. *(circled)* Take a shower first thing in the morning.
    B. Take a shower several times a day, after tennis or swimming.
    C. Take a leisurely bath.

12. **I have help in my home:**
    A. *(circled)* Never.
    B. Once or twice a week.
    C. Full time.
    Okay, occasionally.

13. **I put myself together:**
    A. *(circled)* To please myself.
    B. To suit my life-style.
    C. To please my man.
    A and C.

14. **I work:**
    A. Nine to five at a regular job.
    B. You think taking care of the kids isn't full-time work?
    C. Flexible hours or not at all.

15. **My fingernails:**
    A. Are manicured by me.
    B. *(circled)* Are kept short and neat for simplicity.
    C. I have done weekly.

16. **When it comes to athletics:**
    A. Weekends are the only time I have for recreational sports.
    B. *(circled)* I'd only be more active if I were training for the Olympics.
    C. I don't sweat.
    I work three to five times a week.

17. **If I have a little extra money to splurge with, I:**
    A. Buy something I need.
    B. Get something for the kids.
    C. *(circled)* Buy something wonderful I've been dying to have.

18. **My idea of the perfect vacation would be to:**
    A. Travel to the major cities of Europe.
    B. Go hiking and backpacking.
    C. Escape to a spa.
    go to Hawaii

19. **My bedtime is:**
    A. After the 11:00 P.M. news.
    B. *(circled)* Early, after an exhausting day.
    C. Whenever the party's over.

20. **If I could sum up my beauty routine simply, I would say it's:**
    A. Sensible.
    B. Practical.
    C. Time-consuming.
    Whatever I'm in the mood for

Jose says:
Lisa's hair has lots of fullness on top, to take away from her wide jawline, and bangs, to accentuate her beautiful blue eyes. This wild and messy and sexy look is easy to do. Lisa is very active, and the length of her hair allows her to style it in many ways.

Goldie Hawn

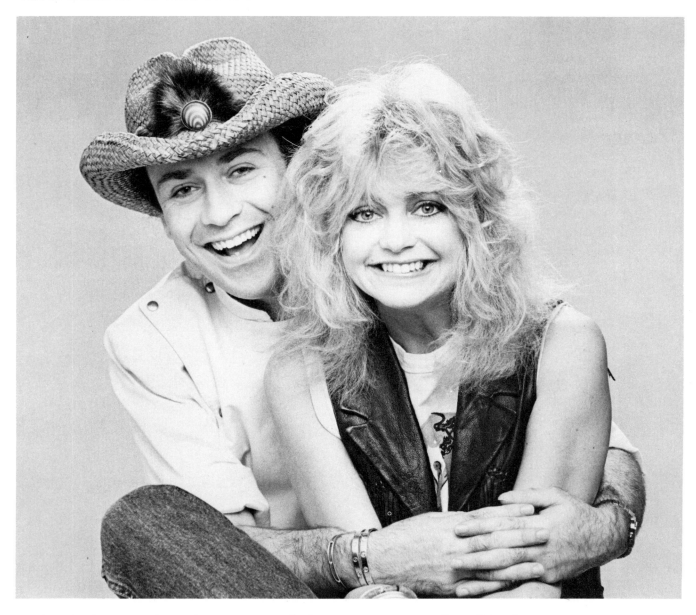

Gosh, I don't remember who recommended Jose to me—one of my friends. Anyway, someone did, and I went to him. He cut and shaped my hair until I was happy, and I've never been happy with a stylist before. I'm not nervous when I'm sitting in his chair; I trust him completely. And it's really difficult for me to go to the hairdresser and sit and not be nervous. If I knew how to cut hair, I think I'd have the scissors in my hand.

Jose likes women. That comes through. And he works well with them.

Usually I come to him in a complete state of confusion, and we work together. I have ideas about my hair. I push my hair around on my head and hold it up and around, and we talk and work things out. I don't believe in bringing in pictures. They're tough to work with. I've done it enough to know they don't help.

Jose and the guy who does my hair on my films are the only people I let touch my hair. If anyone else comes near me, I get crazy. I like my hair a certain way—not too done . . . tousled. I don't care so much about face shape or any of those things; I care about its feeling right to me. And Jose helps me feel right.

JOSE EBER'S LIFE-STYLE QUIZ

Goldie Hawn

1. **When I wake up in the morning:**
   A. I look at the alarm clock and panic. I'm already late.
   (B.) Who needs an alarm clock? I'm up with the birds, or the kids, and ready to go.
   C. I roll over and go back to sleep for another half hour because last night really was a bit too much.

2. **My regular morning routine:**
   (A.) Takes no more than half an hour because I'm so busy.
   B. Is postponed until later in the day, because I'm out the door for tennis or carpool.
   C. Depends on what I'm doing during the day and what's cooking for the upcoming evening.

3. **When I look in the mirror each morning I:**
   A. Wish I had time to do something about what I see.
   (B.) Splash cold water on my face and check the condition of my skin.
   C. Study each line, blemish, and soft spot mercilessly, until I'm satisfied I know exactly how to best care for what I've seen.

4. **First thing in the morning, my hair:**
   A. Needs a wash and blow-dry.
   (B.) Kind of falls into place, because my haircut is easy to care for.
   C. Is almost perfect, because I just had it done yesterday.

5. **My hair:**
   A. Gets cut whenever I'm in the mood or can't do a thing with it.
   (B.) Needs to be cut every four–six weeks; otherwise it's unmanageable.
   C. Is long to allow me to manage a variety of hairstyles depending on my needs so I just make sure the ends are trimmed frequently.

6. **My hair color:**
   A. Is something I've experimented with myself.
   B. Yuck! Put chemicals in my hair with chemicals?
   C. Is done at the beauty shop every six weeks.

   None. I don't color my hair. It's never been permed. It is my natural color.

7. **The colors I wear most frequently are:**
   A. Neutrals that mix well in the business world: navy, burgundy, cream, and things that are "safe."
   (B.) Bright colors, I love 'em.
   C. Whatever the fashion mavens say.

   B. "I guess I'm not very conscious of colors — I just wear what I want."

8. **For a purse, I usually carry:**
   (A.) One good all-purpose bag that goes with all my clothes.
   B. Something fun and inexpensive that holds all the junk I carry around.
   C. Whatever matches my clothes.

9. **The hair appliances I rely on include:**
   (A.) A round brush and blow-dryer.
   B. I have all kinds of stuff, but I never use it.
   C. Electric rollers, hairpins, combs, clips, curling iron, crimper, dryers, and brushes.

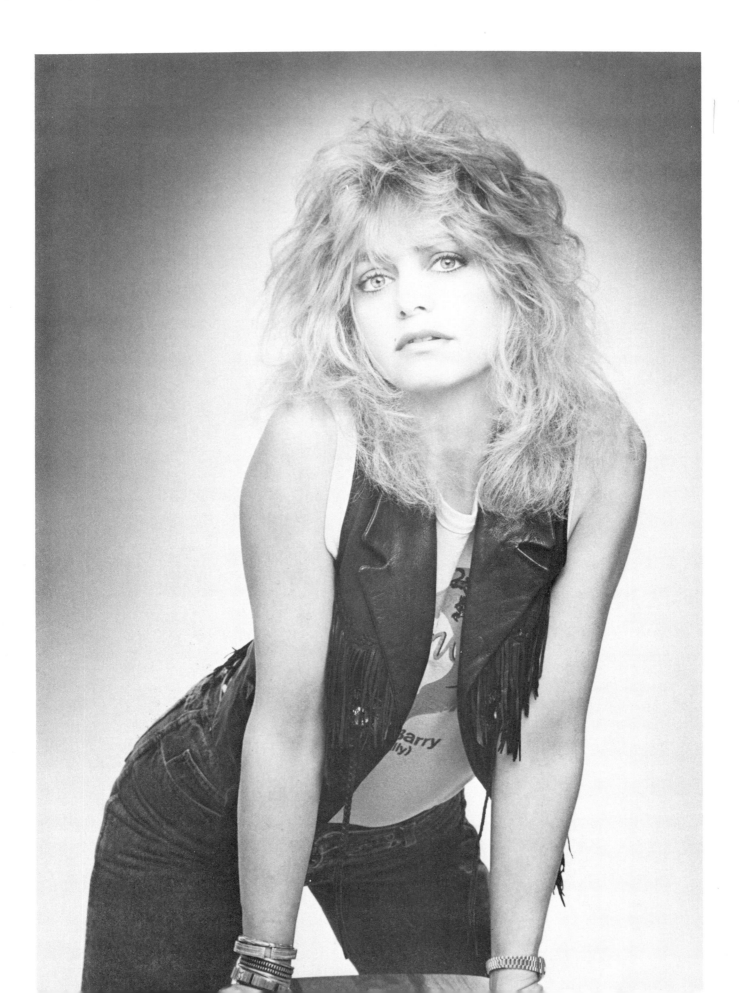

10. **For breakfast, I:**
    A. Grab something on the way to work or eat at my desk
    B. (Have cold cereal and fruit.
    C. Eat a light meal if I'm dieting or a little more if I'm having a late lunch.

11. **When I bathe, I:**
    A. (Take a shower first thing in the morning.
    B. Take a shower several times a day, after tennis or swimming.
    C. Take a leisurely bath.

12. **I have help in my home:**
    A. Never.
    B. Once or twice a week.
    C. (Full time.

13. **I put myself together:**
    A. (To please myself.
    B. To suit my life-style.
    C. To please my man.

14. **I work:**
    A. Nine to five at a regular job.
    B. You think taking care of the kids isn't full-time work?
    C. Flexible hours or not at all.

15. **My fingernails:**
    A. Are manicured by me.

B. (Are kept short and neat for simplicity.
C. I have done weekly.

I never do them my nails are really a mess. Don't look

16. **When it comes to athletics:**
    A. (Weekends are the only time I have for recreational sports.
    B. I'd only be more active if I were training for the Olympics.
    C. I don't sweat.

17. **If I have a little extra money to splurge with, I:**
    A. Buy something I need.
    B. Get something for the kids.
    C. (Buy something wonderful I've been dying to have.

18. **My idea of the perfect vacation would be to:**
    A. Travel to the major cities of Europe.
    B. (Go hiking and backpacking.
    C. Escape to a spa.

19. **My bedtime is:**
    A. (After the 11:00 P.M. news.
    B. Early, after an exhausting day.
    C. Whenever the party's over.

20. **If I could sum up my beauty routine simply, I would say it's:**
    A. Sensible.
    B. (Practical.
    C. Time-consuming.

Jose says:
Goldie has enormous eyes and a long neck, so she needs soft, messy hair to frame her face. The bangs are not a must, but I like them. She has a light body wave for fullness at certain angles, to balance her face. The layers make her hair easy to care for—she doesn't even need a brush—but there is enough length and body so she can smooth out her hair and glamorize her look for special occasions. This is a hairstyle that Goldie can do anything with if she wants to.

Suzy Kalter

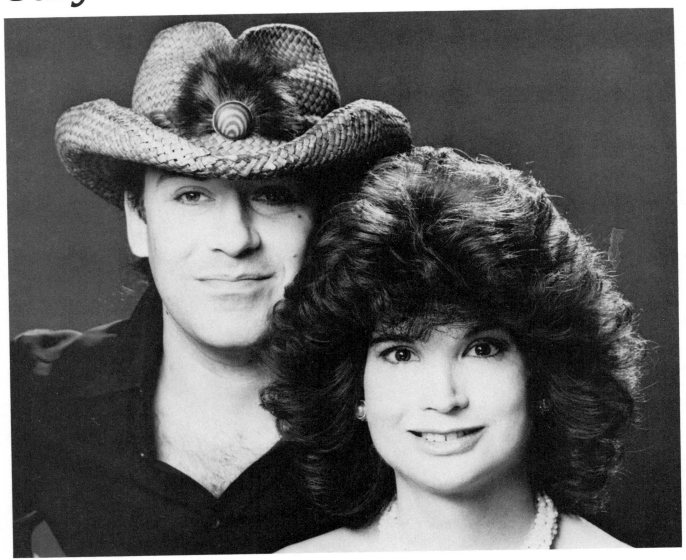

Suzy Kalter is a journalist, an author, and a mother, who has about an hour each morning to get up, shower, do her hair and makeup, get dressed, and play with her son before she goes out to work. Sometimes she sits at a desk and writes all day, but usually she runs around, doing three or four different things: she may write in the morning, go out to conduct an interview, have a lunch date, go to a photographic shooting or a meeting at a studio in connection with another project, and then return to her office or go home to get her son, then make a quick trip to the grocery store with him. Because every day is different and her schedule is so erratic, she must have one look that will last all day and be appropriate for any occasion.

Suzy feels that her biggest problem with her beauty routine is not having the time to do the things that might make her look better. She likes to have her hair styled with hot rollers, but says they are out of the question except for special occasions. She's doesn't even take the time to fully blow-dry her hair! She actually wants to snap her fingers and *voilà*, be gorgeous—presto—but hasn't figured out how to do that yet.

She is a true Life-style Green—she does her hair color herself, never takes time for extra conditioning, and has her hairstyle changed on a whim rather than a schedule. She has a very wide jawline and needs to have soft hair framing it, but she gets impatient or bored with her hair and often has it cut too short for her face. She still believes that short hair is easier than medium-length for her, but finally I am getting her to grow it out longer.

JOSE EBER'S LIFE-STYLE QUIZ

Suzy Kalter

1. **When I wake up in the morning:**
   A. I look at the alarm clock and panic. I'm already late.
   B. Who needs an alarm clock? I'm up with the birds, or the kids, and ready to go.
   C. I roll over and go back to sleep for another half hour because last night really was a bit too much.

2. **My regular morning routine:**
   A. Takes no more than half an hour because I'm so busy.
   B. Is postponed until later in the day, because I'm out the door for tennis or carpool.
   C. Depends on what I'm doing during the day and what's cooking for the upcoming evening.

3. **When I look in the mirror each morning I:**
   A. Wish I had time to do something about what I see.
   B. Splash cold water on my face and check the condition of my skin.
   C. Study each line, blemish, and soft spot mercilessly, until I'm satisfied I know exactly how to best care for what I've seen.

4. **First thing in the morning, my hair:**
   A. Needs a wash and blow-dry.
   B. Kind of falls into place, because my haircut is easy to care for.
   C. Is almost perfect, because I just had it done yesterday.

5. **My hair:**
   A. Gets cut whenever I'm in the mood or can't do a thing with it.
   B. Needs to be cut every four–six weeks; otherwise it's unmanageable.
   C. Is long to allow me to manage a variety of hairstyles depending on my needs so I just make sure the ends are trimmed frequently.

6. **My hair color:**
   A. Is something I've experimented with myself.
   B. Yuck! Ruin my hair with chemicals?
   C. Is done at the beauty shop every six weeks.

7. **The colors I wear most frequently are:**
   A. Neutrals that mix well in the business world: navy, burgundy, cream, and things that are "safe."
   B. Bright colors, I love 'em.
   C. Whatever the fashion mavens say is "in," as long as it's also flattering to my skin tones.

8. **For a purse, I usually carry:**
   A. One good all-purpose bag that goes with all my clothes.
   B. Something fun and inexpensive that holds all the junk I carry around.
   C. Whatever matches my clothes.

9. **The hair appliances I rely on include:**
   A. A round brush and blow-dryer.
   B. I have all kinds of stuff, but I never use it.
   C. Electric rollers, hairpins, combs, clips, curling iron, crimper, dryers, and brushes.

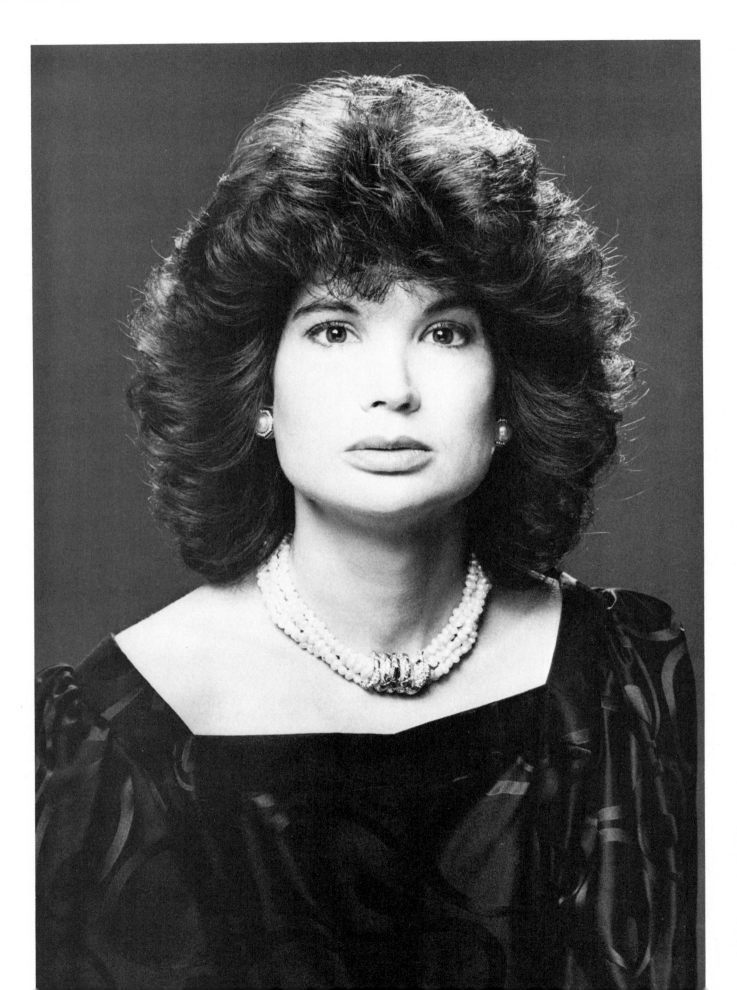

10. **For breakfast, I:**
    A. Grab something on the way to work or eat at my desk

    [handwritten: Have cold breakfast and usually I eat a light meal but I'm dying for a little more if I'm having a lunch at the coffee shop across or a from my office breakfast meeting.]

11. **When I bathe, I:**
    A. Take a shower first thing in the morning.
    B. Take a shower several times a day, after tennis or swimming.
    C. Take a leisurely bath.

    [handwritten: And have a bath at night with my son.]

12. **I have help in my home:**
    A. Never.
    B. Once or twice a week.
    C. Full time.

    [handwritten: She takes care of the baby.]

13. **I put myself together:**
    A. To please myself.
    B. To suit my life-style.

    [handwritten: I'll dress myself to please myself when my child is a little older. Now I have to be chic but practical.]

14. **I work:**
    A. Nine to five at a regular job.
    B. You think taking care of the kids isn't full-time work?
    C. Flexible hours or not at all.

15. **My fingernails:**
    A. Are manicured by me.
    B. Are kept short and neat for simplicity.
    C. I have done weekly.

16. **When it comes to athletics:**
    A. Weekends are the only time I have for recreational sports.
    B. I'd only be more active if I were training for the Olympics.
    C. I don't sweat.

17. **If I have a little extra money to splurge with, I:**
    A. Buy something I need.
    B. Get something for the kids.
    C. Buy something wonderful I've been dying to have.

    [handwritten: It's really B and C. I spend a lot of time at Toys R Us.]

18. **My idea of the perfect vacation would be to:**
    A. Travel to the major cities of Europe.
    B. Go hiking and backpacking.
    C. Escape to a spa.

19. **My bedtime is:**
    A. After the 11:00 P.M. news.
    B. Early, after an exhausting day.
    C. Whenever the party's over.

20. **If I could sum up my beauty routine simply, I would say it's:**
    A. Sensible.
    B. Practical.
    C. Time-consuming.

Jose says:
For Suzy, to take away from her wide jawline and narrow temples, I cut her hair so that there's a lot of it framing the eyes, to give the illusion of the perfect face shape. She also has a long neck, so the hair can fill in there. When her hair is full, she looks perfect. I like this easy-care hairdo, because Suzy is a busy woman, with a job and a child, and she has no time to fuss. Her hair is layered to give her some height and to make the curl last all day. She can finger-style her hair if she is in a hurry, and let it dry naturally, because she has some natural wave, or she can use the electric rollers for a more sophisticated look.

Sally Kellerman

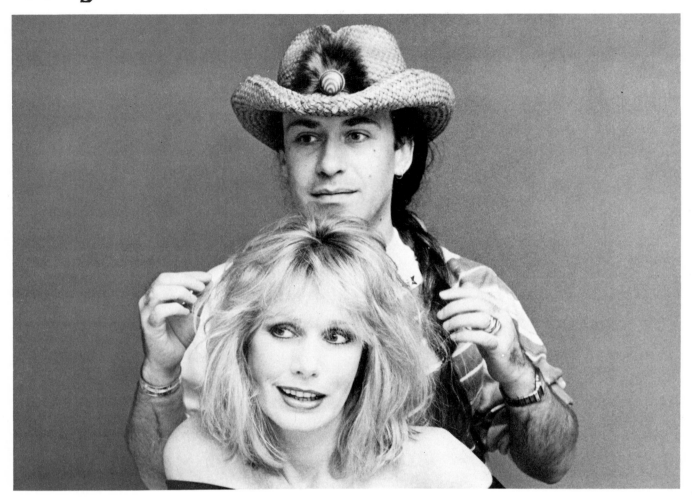

I am my hair. It's my most neurotic area, so when my hair is great, I feel great, like I'm on top of the world. When my hair isn't working, I'm in the dumps. But if my hair looks good, other things about my appearance aren't so important. I like to think that when I put on my makeup I look terrific, but it doesn't matter as much as the hair.

And Jose gives me the kind of haircut that makes me feel wonderful. I have thin, fine hair, and nobody cuts it like Jose. The cut is everything. I don't even have to curl my hair except on special occasions or when I want to. With this cut, even when my hair is wet and tangled, it looks better than it ever did before.

I met Jose a couple of years ago, when I actually went to interview a hairstylist. I thought, "I'm grown up now," so I decided to interview stylists to find one I liked. My regular hairstylist had moved to New York, and I was in a dead panic. I didn't know who Jose was and I had never heard of him, but someone recommended him to me, so I went to see him and about four others. All the others said they thought they'd give me a trim. I walked into Jose's and saw some people with really wild hair, sort of bushy and unkept. Then I saw Jose, and he was wearing a cowboy hat and had a long ponytail, and I said, "Oh, hi," because I didn't know what else to say. Immediately he told me he'd cut off the whole front part of my hair, chop this, and do that, and finally I thought, "Oh, hell, I'll go with him; I can always buy a wig." I wanted to do something daring.

He gave me a great cut, and I was thrilled. After the whole thing was over, I found out he cut Ali and Farrah and Cher's hair, and I felt like a fool. It was so silly, but I didn't know who he was and I thought I was really doing a brave thing. But I knew he'd either ruin me or make me.

JOSE EBER'S LIFE-STYLE QUIZ

Sally Kellerman

1. When I wake up in the morning:
A. I look at the alarm clock and panic. I'm already late.
B. Who needs an alarm clock? I'm up with the birds so the kids are ready to...
C. I roll over and go back to sleep for another half hour because last night really was a bit too much.

my husband watches it and we have an alarm clock in it so that when it goes off we can go back to sleep for a little while.

2. My regular morning routine:
A. Takes no more than half an hour because I'm so busy.
B. Is postponed until later in the day, because I'm out the door for tennis or carpool.
C. Depends on what I'm doing during the day and what's coming for the upcoming events.

I get up and go sit at the piano looking like the subject for the christmas pasty. Then then I go to the piano without makeup or anything and my face has goop in it. Then I go shower.

3. When I look in the mirror I:
A. Wish I had time to do something about what I see.
B. Splash cold water on my face and check the condition of my skin.
C. Study each line, blemish, and soft spot mercilessly, until I'm satisfied I know exactly how to best care for what I've seen.

4. First thing in the morning, my hair:
A. Needs a wash and blow-dry.
B. Kind of falls into place because my haircut is easy to manage.
C. Is almost perfect, because I had that done yesterday.

I have a fabulous cut and it would be B my hair could fall into place, except that I sleep with several pounds of vaseline, so I have to wash my hair

5. My hair:
A. Gets cut whenever I'm in the mood or can't do a thing with it.
B. Needs to be cut every four–six weeks; otherwise it's unmanageable.
C. Is long to allow me to manage a variety of hairstyles depending on my needs so I just make sure the ends are trimmed frequently.

6. My hair color:
A. Is something I've experimented with myself.
B. Yuck! Ruin my hair with chemicals?
C. Is done at the beauty shop every six weeks.

7. The colors I wear most frequently are:
A. Neutrals that mix well in the business world: navy, burgundy, cream, and things that are "safe."
B. Bright colors, I love 'em.
C. Whatever the fashion mavens say is "in," as long as it's also flattering to my skin tones.

I wear whatever color I feel like.

8. For a purse, I usually carry:
A. One good all-purpose bag that goes with all my clothes.
B. Something big and inexpensive that holds all the items I carry around.
C. Whatever matches my clothes.

When I go to meetings or lunches, I use one of my fantastic bags.

9. The hair appliances I rely on include:
A. A round brush and blow-dryer.
B. I have all kinds of stuff, but never use it.
C. Electric rollers, hairpins, combs, curling iron, crimper, dryers, and brushes.

Wire brush, hair dryer, and three foam curlers.

119

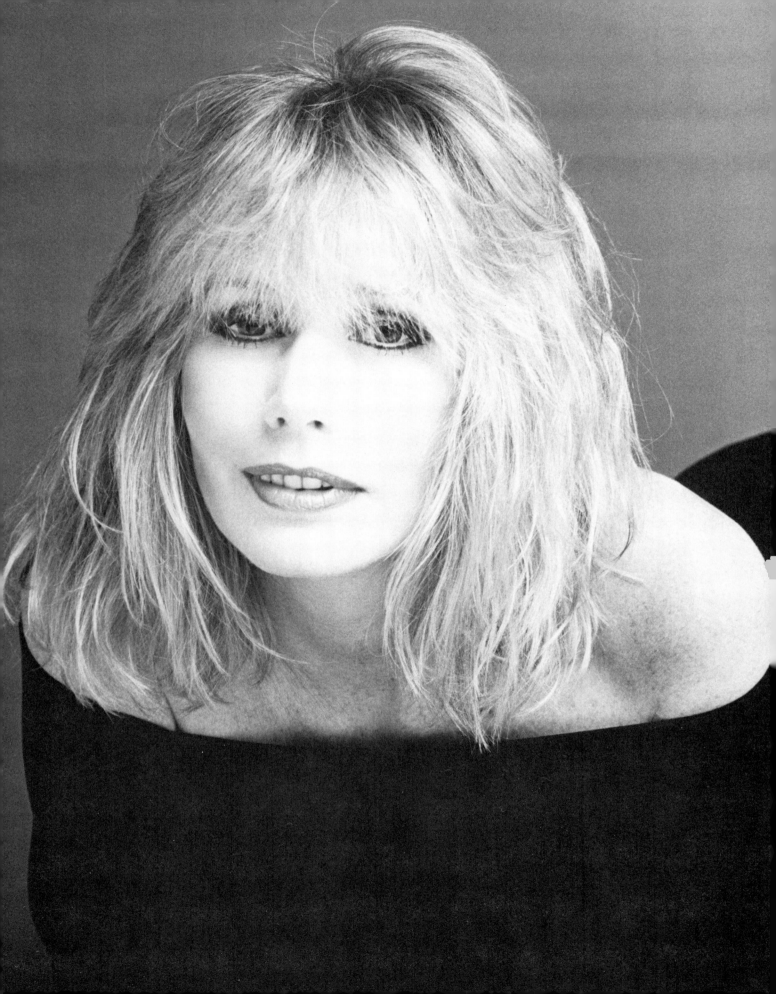

10. **For breakfast, I:**
    A. Grab something on the way to work or eat at my desk
    B. Have cold cereal and fruit.
    C. Eat a light meal if I'm dieting for a little more if I'm having a late lunch.

    I eat every thing I can get my hands on, I don't eat and then a lunch.

11. **When I bathe, I:**
    A. Take a shower first thing in the morning.
    B. Take a shower several times a day, after tennis or swimming.
    C. Take a leisurely bath.

    I take as few showers a day as I can.

12. **I have help in my home:**
    A. Never.
    B. Once or twice a week.
    C. Full time.

13. **I put myself together:**
    A. To please myself
    B. To suit my life-style.
    C. To please my man.

    comfort is the key and I like to please my husband every year he has more influence on my choice of clothes.

14. **I work:**
    A. Nine to five at a regular job.
    B. You think taking care of the kids isn't full-time work?
    C. Flexible hours or not at all.

15. **My fingernails:**
    A. Are manicured by me.

    I always do my nails at the last minute when I go out to sing they're usually still wet.

    B. Are kept short and neat for simplicity.
    C. I have done weekly.

16. **When it comes to athletics:**
    A. Weekends are the only time I have for recreational sports.
    B. I'd only be more active if I were training for the Olympics.
    C. I don't sweat.

    I run and swim

17. **If I have a little extra money to splurge with, I:**
    A. Buy something I need.
    B. Get something for the kids.
    C. Buy something wonderful I've been dying to have.

18. **My idea of the perfect vacation would be to:**
    A. Travel to the major cities of Europe.
    B. Go hiking and backpacking.
    C. Escape to a spa.

19. **My bedtime is:**
    A. After the 11:00 P.M. news.
    B. Early, after an exhausting day.
    C. Whenever the party's over.

20. **If I could sum up my beauty routine simply, I would say it's:**
    A. Sensible.
    B. Practical.
    C. Time-consuming.

    my makeup and hairstyle are simple, but I like to think I'm stunning when I finish.

Jose says:
Sally has an incredible bone structure, and the hair is cut to show off the cheekbones. Her hair is almost all one length, with bangs that are cut on an angle to show her eyes and her bones. She does not need volume in her hair, so it can be blunt-cut and fall naturally.

Victoria Principal

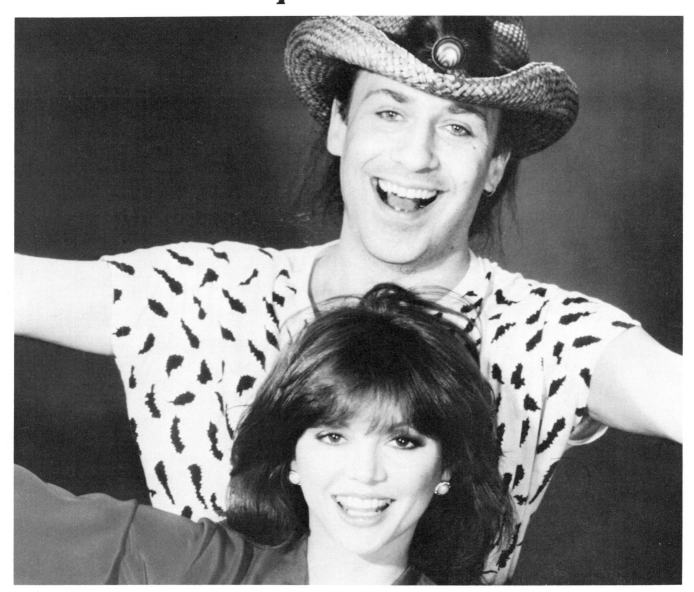

I had been complaining that I was bored with my hair and I didn't think it was as flattering as it could be, and a friend took me by the hand and actually walked me into Jose's. I felt an immediate rapport with Jose, and I don't mean professional. I knew we'd work well together and become friends.

I think that Jose's attention and affection are what keep his clients happy. He's more than good; he really cares. And the encouragement that I've gotten from him when he's doing my hair has affected other areas of my life. When he gave my hair a new image, he gave me a new image, and that affected how I felt about myself, how I dressed, and how I acted. I really began to feel that I was sexier. It's not that I started showing more flesh, but an internal metamorphosis occurred, because of an external factor—a haircut.

I'm really careful about my hair. My skin and my hair are never exposed to direct sunlight—it can change your hair color. I eat well-balanced meals, for my hair, my nails, my mind, and body. I steam my hair in the shower every morning for ten or fifteen minutes before I wash and I condition it. I also use a heavy conditioner whenever I need it. I don't have any specific beauty night; I just answer the call of my body. I believe in preventive conditioning. I don't wait until I need it. That's why I say my beauty look is sensible but time-consuming.

JOSE EBER'S LIFE-STYLE QUIZ   *Victoria Principal*

1. **When I wake up in the morning:**
   - (A.) I look at the alarm clock and panic. I'm already late.
   - B. Who needs an alarm clock? I'm up with the birds, or the kids, and ready to go.
   - C. I roll over and go back to sleep for another half hour because last night really was a bit too much.

2. **My regular morning routine:**
   - A. Takes no more than half an hour because I'm so busy.
   - B. Is postponed until later in the day, because I'm out the door for tennis or carpool.
   - (C.) Depends on what I'm doing during the day and what's cooking for the upcoming evening.

3. **When I look in the mirror each morning I:**
   - A. Wish I had time to do something about what I see.
   - (B.) Splash cold water on my face and check the condition of my skin.
   - C. Study each line, blemish, and soft spot mercilessly, until I'm satisfied I know exactly how to best care for what I've seen.

   B and C

4. **First thing in the morning, my hair:**
   - (A.) Needs a wash and blow-dry.
   - B. Kind of falls into place, because my haircut is easy to care for.
   - C. Is almost perfect, because I just had it done yesterday.

5. **My hair:**
   - A. Gets cut whenever I'm in the mood or can't do a thing with it.
   - (B.) Needs to be cut every four–six weeks; otherwise it's unmanageable.
   - C. Is long to allow me to manage a variety of hairstyles depending on my needs so I just make sure the ends are trimmed frequently.

6. **My hair color:**
   - A. Is something I've experimented with myself.   *I do it every four weeks, max; every time I'm in love*
   - B. Yuck! Ruin my hair with chemicals?
   - (C.) Is done at the beauty shop every six weeks.

7. **The colors I wear most frequently are:**
   - (A.) Neutrals that mix well in the business world: navy, burgundy, cream, and things that are "safe."
   - B. Bright colors, I love 'em.
   - C. Whatever the fashion mavens say is "in," as long as it's also flattering to my skin tones.

8. **For a purse, I usually carry:**
   - (A.) One good all-purpose bag that goes with all my clothes.
   - B. Something fine and inexpensive that holds all the junk.
   - C. Whatever matches my clothes.

   A and sometimes I carry two bags, one that holds my junk, which stays in the car, and the other to go with what I'm wearing

9. **The hair appliances I rely on include:**
   - (A.) A round brush and blow-dryer.
   - B. I have all kinds of stuff, but I never use it.
   - C. Electric rollers, hairpins, combs, clips, curling iron, crimper, dryers, and brushes.

   And hot curlers

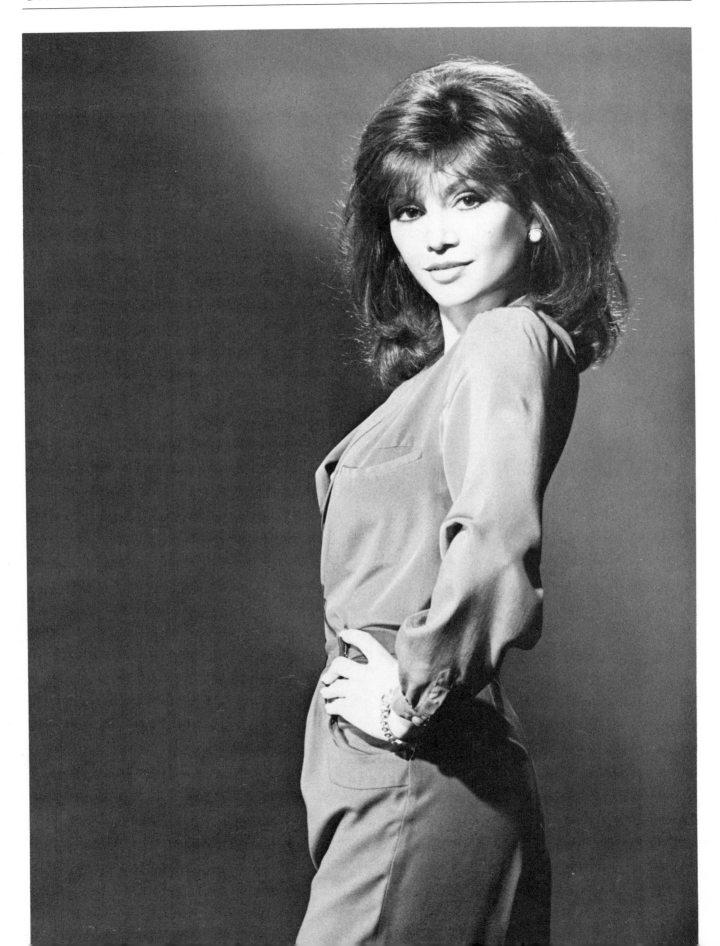

10. For breakfast, I:
   A. Grab something on the way to work, eat at my desk.
   B. Have cold cereal and fruit.
   C. Eat a light meal if I'm dieting.

I eat a big breakfast. I consume small cities. If I'm cut back, dieting I may eat more, but I always eat some breakfast.

11. When I bathe, I:
   A. Take a shower first thing in the morning.
   B. Take a shower several times; after tennis or swimming.
   C. Take a leisurely bath.

But I try to take a bath at the end of the day too.

12. I have help in my home:
   A. Never.
   B. Once or twice a week.
   C. Full time.

13. I put myself together:
   A. To please myself.
   B. To suit my life-style.
   C. To please my man.

A and C

14. I work:
   A. Nine to five at a regular job.
   B. You think taking care of the kids isn't full-time work?
   C. Flexible hours or not at all.

15. My fingernails:
   A. Are manicured by me.

   B. Are kept short and neat for simplicity.
   C. I have done weekly.

16. When it comes to athletics:
   A. Weekends are the only time I have for recreational sports.
   B. I'd only be more active if I were training for the Olympics.
   C. I don't sweat.

I'm very very active on weekends.

17. If I have a little extra money to splurge with, I:
   A. Buy something I need.
   B. Get something for the kids.
   C. Buy something wonderful I've been dying to have.

All of the above.

18. My idea of the perfect vacation would be to:
   A. Travel to the major cities of Europe.
   B. Go hiking and backpacking.
   C. Escape to a spa.

All of them; I like to do as much as possible on vacation.

19. My bedtime is:
   A. After the 11:00 P.M. news.
   B. Early, after an exhausting day.
   C. Whenever the party's over.

B and C

20. If I could sum up my beauty routine simply, I would say it's:
   A. Sensible.
   B. Practical.
   C. Time-consuming.

A and C: it's sensible but time-consuming.

Jose says:
Victoria has a tiny face, and she likes bangs to accentuate her beautiful eyes and mouth. Her hair is very straight, and slightly layered to give some volume on the top. This makes for a younger, sexier look that works with all this mass of Irish Setter hair to balance her tiny face.

125

Sarah Purcell

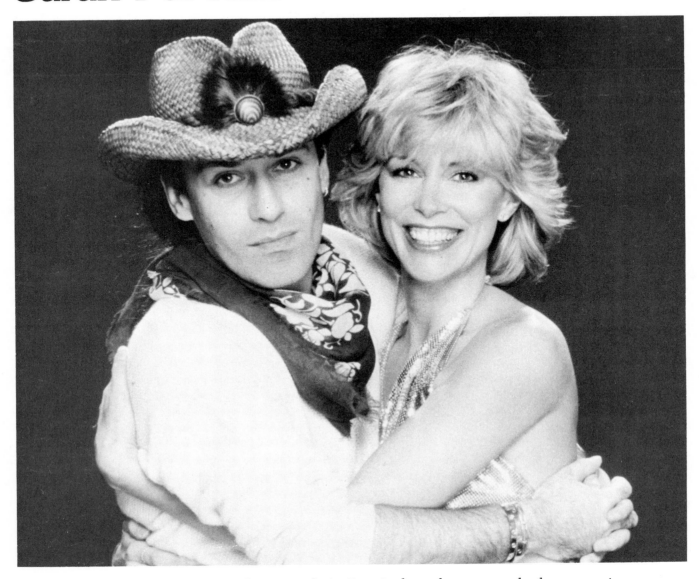

I am the worst when it comes to fixing my hair. Jose is the only person who has ever given me a cut that I can handle. Thanks to him, I can go out in public without having to wear a hat!

I'm the kind of person who is always on the run—while I'm driving to work, I put on half my makeup or have my protein drink for breakfast. I'm not good with hair, and I haven't got the time to fool around with it. Besides, when I'm working, I can be in all kinds of crazy situations that aren't conducive to taking a mirror out of your handbag and plugging in your electric rollers—such as being in the Grand Canyon or on a horse ranch. Once I did an interview on a skyscraper that was in the middle of being built, and there I was, alone with some guys, way up in the wild blue yonder. If you haven't got a good haircut, believe me, this isn't the time to start worrying about whether your curls are hanging in the right place.

My hair's long enough to give me versatility, but I still consider that it's shortish to medium-long, which is easy for my busy life. Jose has given me a new freedom.

JOSE EBER'S LIFE-STYLE QUIZ

Sarah Purcell

1. When I wake up in the morning:
- **(A.)** I look at the alarm clock and panic. I'm already late.
- **B.** Who needs an alarm clock? I'm up with the birds, or the kids, and ready to go.
- **C.** I roll over and go back to sleep for another half hour because last night really was a bit too much.

2. My regular morning routine:
- **A.** Takes no more than half an hour because I'm so busy.
- **(B.)** Is postponed until later in the day, because I'm out the door for tennis or carpool.
- **C.** Depends on what I'm doing during the day and what's cooking for the upcoming evening.

3. When I look in the mirror each morning I:
- **A.** Wish I had time to do something about what I see.
- **(B.)** Splash cold water on my face and check the condition of my skin.
- **C.** Study each line, blemish, and soft spot mercilessly, until I'm satisfied I know exactly how to best care for what I've seen.

It's a combination of A and B.

4. First thing in the morning, my hair:
- **A.** Needs a wash and blow-dry.
- **(B.)** Kind of falls into place, because my haircut's easy to care for.
- **C.** Is almost perfect, because I just had it done yesterday.

And if it falls into place I can give myself a quick spritz with my trusty curling iron.

doesn't fall into place I can give myself my trusty curling iron. I have a comb but I rely on one quick spritz

5. My hair:
- **A.** Gets cut whenever I'm in the mood or can't do a thing with it.
- **(B.)** Needs to be cut every four–six weeks; otherwise it's unmanageable.
- **C.** Is long to allow me to manage a variety of hairstyles depending on my needs. I just make sure the ends are trimmed frequently.

It's four weeks like clockwork or it totally goes overgrown and out of whack.

6. My hair color:
- **A.** Is something I've experimented with myself.
- **B.** Yuck! Ruin my hair with chemicals?
- **(C.)** Is done at the beauty shop every six weeks.

It's also A.

7. The colors I wear most frequently are:
- **A.** Neutrals that mix well in the business world: navy, burgundy, cream, and things that are "safe."
- **B.** Bright colors. I love them.
- **C.** Whatever the fashion magazines say, as long as it's also flattering for my skin tones.
- **D.** *It's mostly A but I have a lot of clothes that fall into different aspects of my work — one on the show, one for me, two different business functions, one for me with my fiancé Peter.*

8. For a purse, I usually carry:
- **(A.)** One good all-purpose bag that goes with all my clothes.
- **B.** Something fun and inexpensive that holds all the junk I carry around.
- **C.** Whatever matches my clothes.

It's A + C, but sometimes I just buy one good bag a year.

9. The hair appliances I rely on include:
- **A.** A round brush and blow-dryer.
- **B.** I have all kinds of stuff, but I never use it.
- **(C.)** Electric rollers, hair curls, combs, clips, curling iron, crimper, dryers, and brushes.

Not all, but of course I'll use everything during of a day.

127

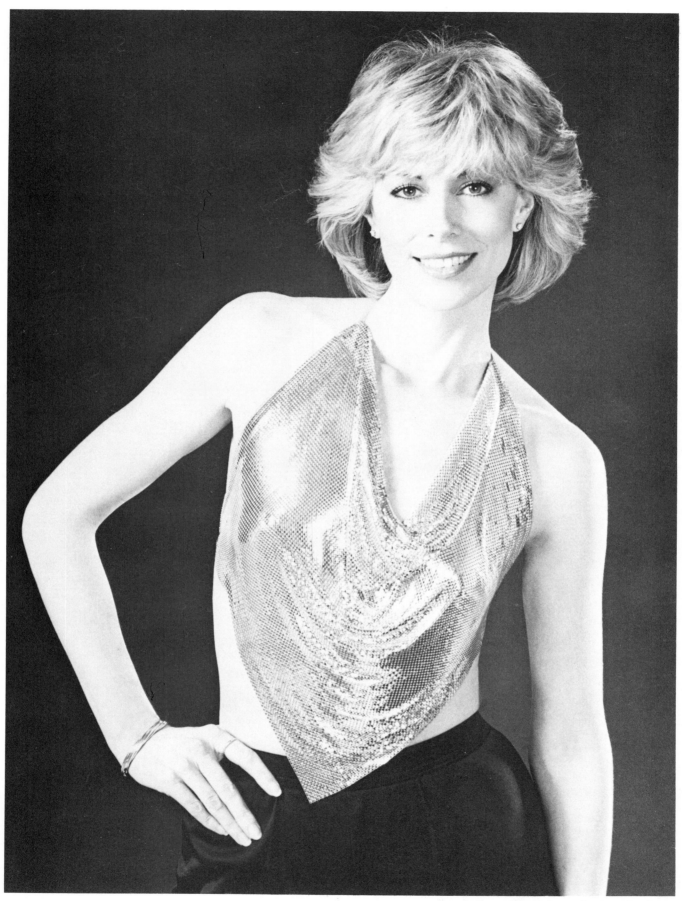

Sarah Purcell's makeup by Carole Shaw.

10. For breakfast, I:
A. Grab something on the way to work or eat at my desk.
B. Have some cereal and fruit.
C. Eat a light meal if I am dieting or a little more if I'm having a late lunch.

I grab a protein drink going out the door and drink it in the car on the way to work

11. When I bathe, I:
A. Take a shower first thing in the morning.
B. Take a shower several times a day, after tennis or swimming.
C. Take a leisurely bath.

12. I have help in my home:
A. Never.
B. Once or twice a week.
C. Full time.

13. I put myself together:
A. To please myself.
B. To suit my lifestyle.
C. To please my man.

all three. I have to suit my lifestyle, but if my man says he hates green, then I won't wear it.

14. I work:
A. Nine to five at a regular job.
B. You think taking care of the kids isn't full-time work?
C. Flexible hours or not at all.

15. My fingernails:
A. Are manicured by me.
B. Are kept short and neat for simplicity.
C. I have done weekly.

all three. I have them done once a month, have my color done, the rest of the time I do them myself.

16. When it comes to athletics:
A. Weekends are the only time I have for recreational sports.
B. I'd only be more active if I were training for the Olympics.
C. I don't sweat.

I jog every day up to about three miles and I have a workout every other day. I play tennis when I can.

17. If I have a little extra money to splurge with, I:
A. Buy something I need.
B. Get something for the kids.
C. Buy something wonderful I've been dying to have.

I'd do both B and C. I keep buying my secretary presents because she's so terrific.

18. My idea of the perfect vacation would be:
A. Travel to the major cities of Europe.
B. Going hiking and backpacking.
C. Escaping to a spa.

this one really depends on what I am. I do this too. I go camping trip with some friends, we're all sort of overgrown Girl Scouts, and I love to go to Europe and I went to a spa once and absolutely loved that!

19. My bedtime is:
A. After the 11:00 P.M. news.
B. Early, after an exhausting day.
C. Whenever the party's over.

After the news I read for an hour.

20. If I could sum up my beauty routine simply, I would say it's:
A. Sensible.
B. Practical.
C. Time-consuming.

and fast too. If I can't do it in ten minutes that's too bad.

Jose says:
Sarah loves change and wants her hairstyle to be different every time she comes to me. Now she has one that is young-looking and funky. She likes bangs, because she has a long face, and the bangs cut that length. She has no perm, because she doesn't need more volume on the top and she has plenty of hair. There are layers cut into the sides, to make her face look a little fuller and to soften the chin line. The hairstyle is also easy to care for, which Sarah needs, because she travels a lot, is on camera often, and needs to have a hairstyle that makes her look good no matter where she is or who she is interviewing . . . and sometimes she gets into crazy interview situations!

Marge Schicktanz

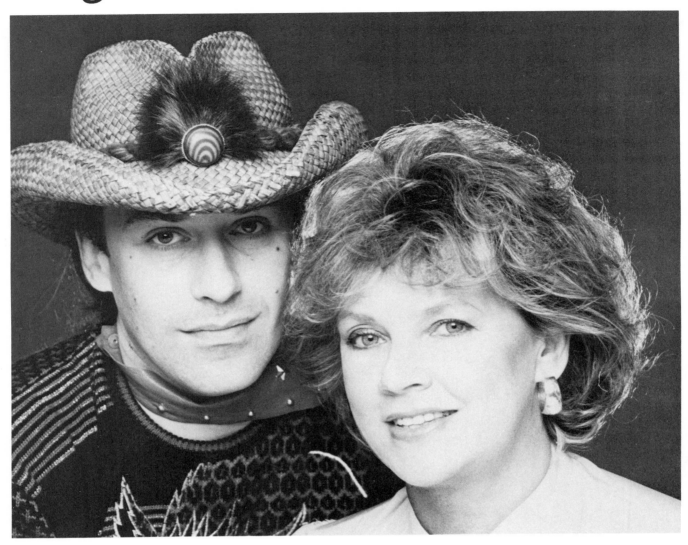

Marge was head of the West Coast commercials department at the William Morris Agency for ten years. Now she's a commercial agent for several big-name celebrities. She works out of her home, but I think she does most of her work at lunch. She likes to group all her appointments together so she can go from one to the other or be at home without having to keep running back and forth.

She is typical of the woman who works for herself with her home as base. She can walk around the house or do her telephone work with her hair in rollers, but once she gets in the car to face the world, she has to look her best. And because she represents so many big stars, she has to look powerful, sophisticated, and glamorous. She needs a hairstyle that will flatter her and won't wilt.

Marge uses electric rollers when she has to, but prefers old-fashioned ones, because they won't damage her hair; and since she has some privacy at home, she can wash her hair, put it in rollers, and do her work while her hair dries naturally. She doesn't damage her hair this way, and still gets the fullness and body it needs to ensure staying power.

JOSE EBER'S LIFE-STYLE QUIZ

Marge Schicktanz

1. **When I wake up in the morning:**
   A. I look at the alarm clock and panic. I'm already late.
   B. Who needs an alarm clock? I'm up with the birds, or the kids, and ready to go.
   C. I roll over and go back to sleep for another half-hour because last night really was a bit too much.

   D. I deliberately set the clock ahead so I can go back to sleep.

2. **My regular morning routine:**
   (A.) Takes no more than half an hour because I'm so busy.
   B. Is postponed until later in the day, because I'm out the door for tennis or carpool.
   C. Depends on what I'm doing during the day and what's cooking for the upcoming evening.

3. **When I look in the mirror each morning I:**
   (A.) Wish I had time to do something about what I see.
   B. Splash cold water on my face and check the condition of my skin.
   C. Study each line, blemish, and soft spot mercilessly, until I'm satisfied I know exactly how to best care for what I've seen.

4. **First thing in the morning, my hair:**
   A. Needs a wash and blow-dry.
   B. Kind of falls into place, because my haircut is so sophisticated.
   C. Is almost perfect, because I just had it done yesterday.

   D. Start from scratch even if I said I have it done; my fantasy is to have my hair last all day.

5. **My hair:**
   (A.) Gets cut whenever I'm in the mood or can't do a thing with it.
   B. Needs to be cut every four–six weeks; otherwise it's unmanageable.
   C. Is long to allow me to manage a variety of hairstyles depending on my needs so I just make sure the ends are trimmed frequently.

6. **My hair color:**
   A. Is something I've experimented with myself.
   B. Yuck! Ruin my hair with chemicals?
   (C.) Is done at the beauty shop every six weeks.

   make that irregularly

7. **The colors I wear most frequently are:**
   A. Neutrals that mix well in the business world: navy, burgundy, cream, and things that are "safe."
   (B.) Bright colors, I love 'em.
   C. Whatever the fashion mavens say is "in," as long as it's also flattering to my skin tones.

8. **For a purse, I usually carry:**
   (A.) One good all-purpose bag that goes with all my clothes.
   B. Something fun and inexpensive that holds all the junk I carry around.
   C. Whatever matches my clothes.

9. **The hair appliances I rely on include:**
   A. A round brush and blow-dryer.
   B. I have all kinds of stuff, but I never use it.
   (C.) Electric rollers, hairpins, combs, clips, curling iron, crimper, dryers, and brushes.

   D. Hot rollers or regular rollers

131

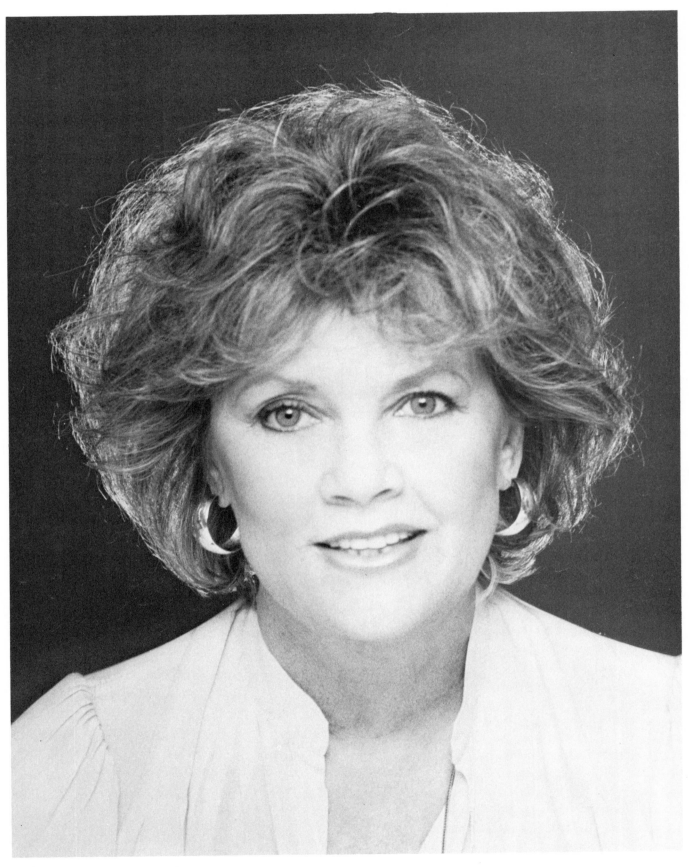

10. **For breakfast, I:**
    A. Grab something on the way to work or eat at my desk.
    B. Have a cold cereal and fruit.
    C. Eat a light meal if I'm dieting or a little more if I'm having a late lunch.

    [handwritten] I don't either. I have eat breakfast. on the road unless I'm on vacation; then a diet powder drink I feel like I've been given a license to eat.

11. **When I bathe:**
    A. Take a shower first thing in the morning.
    B. Take a shower several times a day, after gym or swimming.
    C. Take a leisurely bath. *(C circled)*

    [handwritten] I read the trades while I take a long bubble bath.

12. **I have help in my home:**
    A. Never.
    B. Once or twice a week. *(B circled)*
    C. Full time.

13. **I put myself together:**
    A. To please myself. *(A circled)*
    B. To suit my life-style.
    C. To please my man.

    [handwritten] All of them.

14. **I work:**
    A. Nine to five at a regular job. *(A circled)*
    B. You think taking care of the kids isn't full-time work?
    C. Flexible hours or not at all.

    [handwritten] It's more like 7:30 A.M. to 11:30 P.M.

15. **My fingernails:**
    A. Are manicured by me.
    B. Are kept short and neat for simplicity.
    C. I have done weekly.

    [handwritten] I have porcelains built on.

16. **When it comes to athletics:**
    A. Weekends are the only time I have for recreational sports.
    B. I'd only be more active if I were training for the Olympics.
    C. I don't sweat.
    D. *[handwritten] Every day is different; some days are sporty; others aren't.*

17. **If I have a little extra money to splurge with, I:**
    A. Buy something I need.
    B. Get something for the kids. *(B circled)*
    C. Buy something wonderful I've been dying to have.

18. **My idea of the perfect vacation would be to:**
    A. Travel to the major cities of Europe.
    B. Go hiking and backpacking.
    C. Escape to a spa.
    D. *[handwritten] Scotland to hide far side out with a few trips to London.*

19. **My bedtime is:**
    A. After the 11:00 P.M. news. *(A circled)*
    B. Early, after an exhausting day.
    C. Whenever the party's over.

    [handwritten] A or B, depending.

20. **If I could sum up my beauty routine simply, I would say it's:**
    A. Sensible.
    B. Practical. *(B circled)*
    C. Time-consuming.

Jose says:
Marge has incredibly fine hair and a round face, so she feels better with shorter hair and some fullness on top. Her whole face shows with the hair swept back at the sides and off the forehead, because she has a very good forehead, and this gives the illusion of a longer face. If there were hair all around her face, it would accentuate the roundness, like a picture frame, and this would not be as flattering as her hair is now.

Tina Sinatra

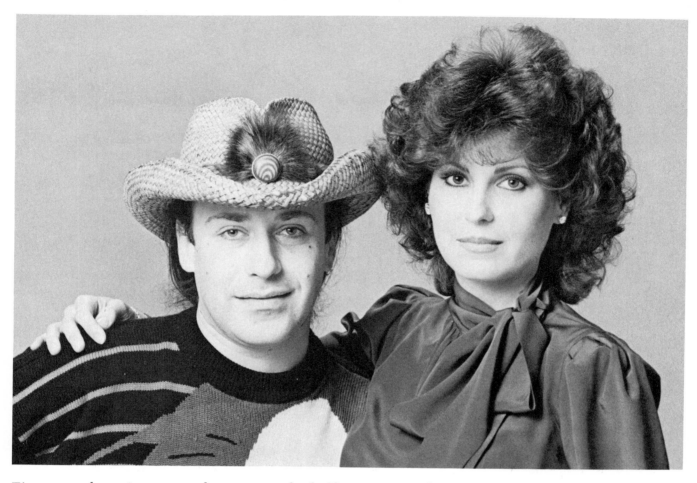

Tina started coming to me about two and a half years ago, when I was recommended to her by a friend, and we've been going great ever since. Tina has a cut that's easy to care for, because she's so busy. She can let it dry naturally, or use hot curlers for a dressier look.

She gets up at about 7:45 or 8:00 A.M. and has coffee in bed. She's in the tub by 8:45. She takes a quick bath, then rinses herself in the shower. She washes her hair every other day. She uses a conditioner while in the shower. On the days when she doesn't wash her hair, she wets it in order to style it. On the weekends she does a heavy conditioning and gives herself a facial.

She can use electric rollers or depend on her perm to help the style to stay. Her cut has to be kept up so the style lasts. Tina's hair grows so fast that it needs to be cut more often than most.

Her life-style is very typical of the working woman's: while she has a little leeway in the morning, because she doesn't have to be at work until 10:00 A.M., she has no more time during the day for her beauty routine or her look. Whatever she does has to last the whole day and into the night, because Tina comes home from work and doesn't have time to change her clothes before going out for dinner. Her hair must last and last and look good!

JOSE EBER'S LIFE-STYLE QUIZ   *Tina Sinatra*

1. **When I wake up in the morning:**
   A. I look at the alarm clock and panic. I'm already late.
   B. Who needs an alarm clock? I'm up with the birds, or the kids, and ready to go.
   (C.) I roll over and go back to sleep for another half hour because last night really was a bit too much.

2. **My regular morning routine:** *the*
   A. Takes no more than half an hour because I'm so busy.
   B. Is postponed until later in the day, because I'm out the door for tennis or carpool.
   C. Depends on what I'm doing during the day and what I'm cooking for the upcoming evening.

   It takes more minutes for the than this to last into but has to last into whole day and evening. into the evening.

3. **When I look in the mirror each morning I:**
   A. Wish I had time to do something about what I see.
   B. Splash cold water on my face and check the condition of my skin.
   C. Study each line, blemish, and soft spot mercilessly, until I'm satisfied I know exactly how to best care for what I've seen.

   D. I sigh.

4. **First thing in the morning, my hair:**
   (A.) Needs a wash and blow-dry.
   B. Kind of falls into place, because my haircut is easy to care for.
   C. Is almost perfect, because I just had it done yesterday.

   A—every other day; I wish I could answer C.

5. **My hair:**
   A. Gets cut whenever I'm in the mood or can't do a thing with it.
   (B.) Needs to be cut every four–six weeks; otherwise it's unmanageable.
   C. Is long to allow *hair* for a variety of hairstyles depending on my need, so I just make sure the ends are trimmed frequently.

   four, never more than three weeks, 'cos it grows real fast.

6. **My hair color:**
   A. Is something I've experimented with myself.
   B. Yuck! Ruin my hair with chemicals?
   C. Is done at the beauty shop every six weeks.

   I've never touched the color—yet.

7. **The colors I wear most frequently are:**
   A. Neutrals that mix well in the business world: navy, burgundy, cream, and things that are "safe."
   (B.) Bright colors, I love 'em.
   C. Whatever the fashion mavens say is "in," as long as it's also flattering to my skin tones.

   Everything but C.

8. **For a purse, I usually carry:**
   (A.) One good all-purpose bag that goes with all my clothes.
   B. Something fun and inexpensive that holds all the junk I carry around.
   C. Whatever matches my clothes.

   Most definitely.

9. **The hair appliances I rely on include:**
   (A.) A round brush and blow-dryer.
   B. I have all kinds of stuff, but I never use it.
   C. Electric rollers, hairpins, combs, clips, curling iron, trimmer, dryers, and brushes.

   brush, hot curlers, and clean hair.

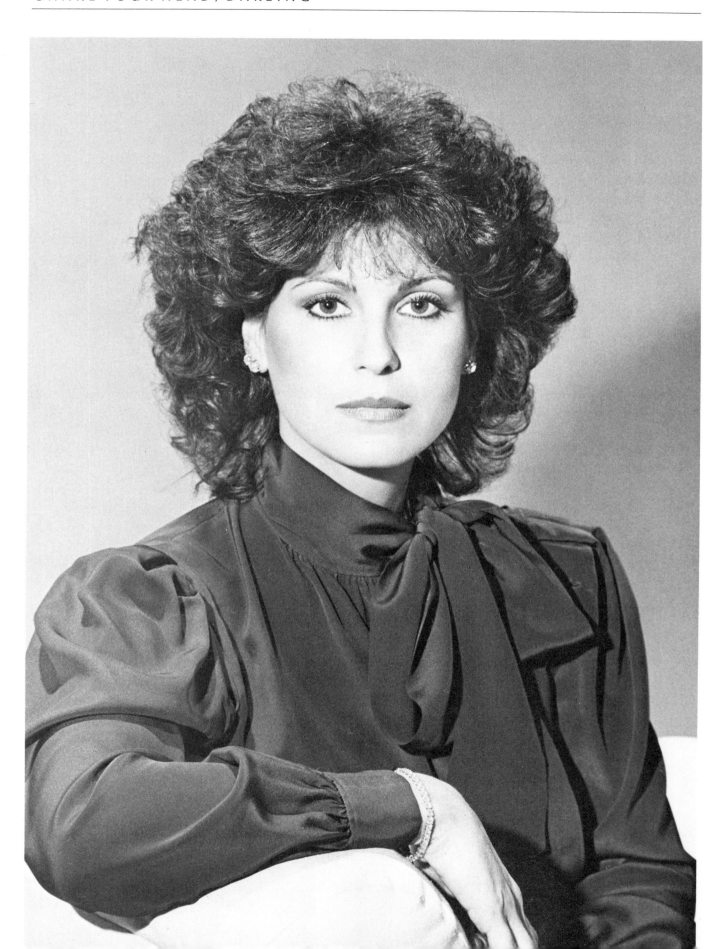

10. **For breakfast, I:**
    A. Grab something on the way to work or eat at my desk
    B. Have cold cereal and fruit.
    C. Eat a light meal if I'm dieting or a little more if I'm having a late lunch.

    I don't eat breakfast.

11. **When I bathe, I:**
    (A.) Take a shower first thing in the morning.
    B. Take a shower several times a day, after tennis or swimming.
    C. Take a leisurely bath.

    I take a not leisurely bath first in the morning.

12. **I have help in my home:**
    A. Never.
    B. Once or twice a week.
    (C.) Full time.

13. **I put myself together:**
    (A.) To please myself.
    B. To suit my life-style.
    C. To please my man.

    I think they all overlap, in varying degrees.

14. **I work:**
    (A.) Nine to five at a regular job.
    B. You think taking care of the kids isn't full-time work.
    C. Flexible hours or not at all.

    It's more like ten to six.

15. **My fingernails:**
    A. Are manicured by me.
    B. Are kept short and neat for simplicity.
    (C.) I have done weekly.

    But I do keep them short because I'm a Klutz.

16. **When it comes to athletics:**
    (A.) Weekends are the only time I have for recreational sports.
    B. I'd only be more active if I were training for the Olympics.
    C. I don't sweat.

17. **If I have a little extra money to splurge with, I:**
    A. Buy something I need.
    B. Get something for the kids.
    (C.) Buy something wonderful I've been dying to have.

18. **My idea of the perfect vacation would be to:**
    A. Travel to the major cities of Europe.
    B. Go hiking and backpacking.
    C. Escape to a spa.

    None of these — maybe Hawaii — I'd like to be on a beach where there's no telephones.

19. **My bedtime is:**
    A. After the 11:00 P.M. news.
    B. Early, after an exhausting day.
    C. Whenever the party's over.

    all three.

20. **If I could sum up my beauty routine simply, I would say it's:**
    A. Sensible.
    (B.) Practical.
    C. Time-consuming.

Jose says:
Tina is a very attractive woman, who needs a hairdo that is easy to take care of, because she is so busy. She has a permanent and a good haircut, so that the style can last all day and into the night. The bangs and the short sides give her an up-to-date look that is becoming and free. Her face is the kind that lets her wear any hairstyle.

Brenda Vaccaro

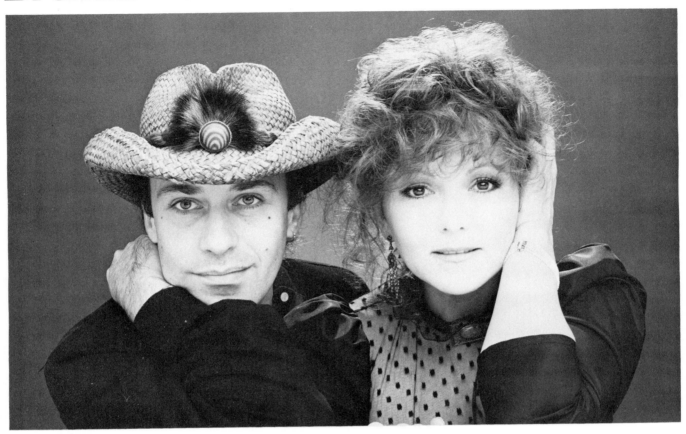

When I met Jose, I saw that he had a long braid, and immediately I thought, "Thank God he's got a braid; that means he respects long hair." So his look didn't upset me at all. I had basically stopped going to hairdressers. I hate them all, especially the whole Beverly Hills scene. But after I met Jose, I called and made an appointment right away. When I got there, we laughed and giggled and he cut off all my hair right then and there. All of it. So much for his respecting long hair!

I had walked in looking like Mrs. Green Hulk. I had perm damage. I had color damage that only Clairol could save. Jose cut off all my hair so it could be born again with him. My hair was short for about a year, until we got it in good condition, and then it grew.

Listen, honey, I've been a professional actress since 1961, and I've been to every fancy hairdresser in the world. They all want to do their thing to you, and after a haircut, from one of them, I'd go home and cry. It's a big deal, psychologically, to have your hair touched. When someone gets hold of you and imposes his will on you, and you have nothing to do with it, it's very, very difficult.

When I walked out of Jose's I felt peaceful. I looked pretty. Even though my hair was short, it had life. The style wasn't extreme. Jose had a sense of what would be pretty on me. He didn't just do what he did to everyone else. Jose gives me my own look, and that's what's important.

You know, a hairdresser has no magic for you. No one can make you look any better than who you are. Makeup and hair can make you look like someone else, but that's not what looking good is about. The best thing any woman can do for herself is to find someone who cares about her first and himself second, like Jose. And that's the truth, sweetheart.

JOSE EBER'S LIFE-STYLE QUIZ

Brenda Vaccaro

1. **When I wake up in the morning:**
   A. I look at the alarm clock and panic. I'm already late.
   (B.) Who needs an alarm clock? I'm up with the birds, or the kids, and ready to go.
   C. I roll over and go back to sleep for another half hour because last night really was a bit too much.

2. **My regular morning routine:**
   (A.) Takes no more than half an hour because I'm so busy.
   B. Is postponed until later in the day, because I'm out the door for tennis or carpool.
   C. Depends on what I'm doing during the day and what's cooking for the upcoming evening.

3. **When I look in the mirror each morning I:**
   A. Wish I had time to do something about what I see.
   (B.) Splash cold water on my face and check the condition of my skin. Study each line, blemish, and soft spot mercilessly, until I'm satisfied I know exactly how to take care of what I've seen.

   none of them — I just wash my face and get on with the day, too, I brush my teeth, too!

4. (4.) **First thing in the morning, my hair:**
   A. Needs a wash and blow-dry.
   B. Kind of falls into place, because my haircut is easy to care for.
   C. Is almost perfect, because I just had it done yesterday.

5. **My hair:**
   A. Gets cut whenever I'm in the mood and can't do a thing with it.
   (B.) Needs to be cut every four-six weeks but otherwise it's manageable.
   C. Is long to allow me to manage a variety of hairstyles depending on my needs so I just make sure the ends are trimmed frequently.

   Well, it's B and C and the ends trimmed every month because it's kind of long that's the most complimentary to my face!

6. **My hair color:**
   A. Is something I've experimented with myself.
   (B.) Yuck! Ruin my hair with chemicals.
   C. Is done at the beauty shop every six weeks.

   It's B and C I think I hate highlights and they are absolutely terrible for your hair and that's my final position.

7. **The colors I wear most frequently are:**
   (A.) Neutrals that mix well in the business world: navy, burgundy, cream, and things that are "safe."
   B. Bright colors I dress 'em up. Whatever the fashion mavens say is in, as long as it's also flattering to my skin tone.

   except that right now my hair is colored. change the word "safe" to "classic" please. I like sane colors like black and burgundy not stupid crazy colors.

8. **For a purse, I usually carry:**
   (A.) One good all-purpose bag that goes with all my clothes.
   B. Something fun and inexpensive that holds all the junk I carry around.
   C. Whatever matches my clothes.

9. **The hair appliances I rely on included:**
   A. A round brush, a blow-dryer.
   B. I've tried all kinds of stuff, but in England and...
   (C.) Electric rollers, hairpins, combs, curling iron, crimpers, and brushes.

   I use the blower rollers, a good hairbrush the old-fashioned hairpins I use like your grandmother used to use.

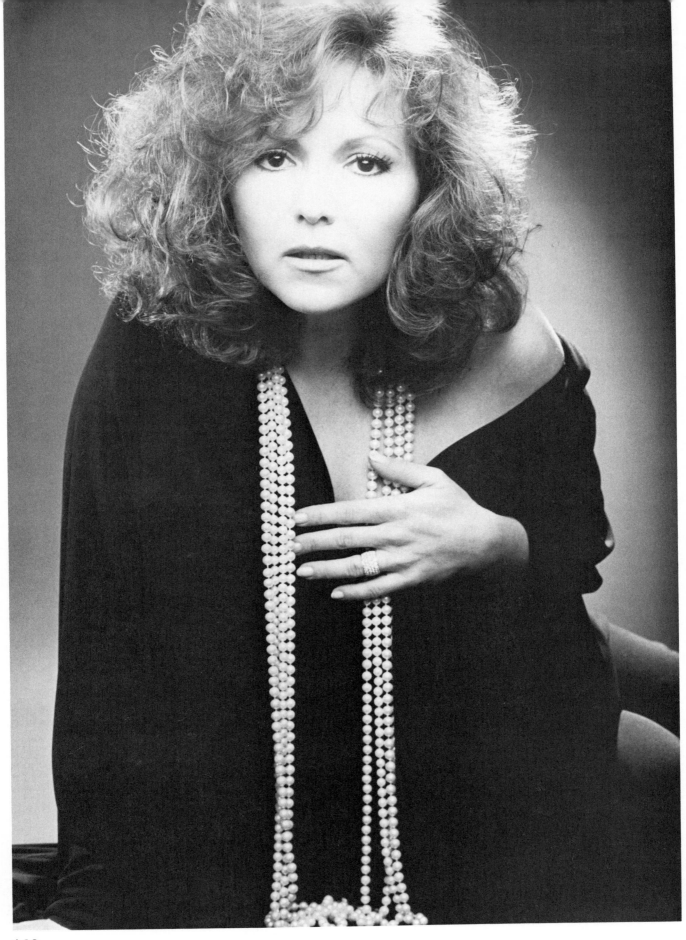

10. For breakfast, I:
- A. Grab something on the way to work or eat at my desk
- B. Have cold cereal and fruit.
- (C.) Eat a light meal if I'm dieting or a little more if I'm having a late lunch.

I'm a bit of both B and C.

11. When I bathe, I:
- A. Take a shower first thing in the morning.
- (B.) Take a shower several times a day, after tennis or swimming.
- C. Take a leisurely bath.

I do all three.

12. I have help in my home:
- A. Never.
- B. Once or twice a week.
- C. Full time.

I have a staff of fourteen, you cutie. No, no, no - I'm only kidding.

13. I put myself together:
- (A.) To please myself.
- B. To suit my life-style.
- C. To please my man.

14. I work:
- A. Nine to five at a regular job.
- B. You think taking care of the kids isn't full-time work?
- C. Flexible hours or not at all.

15. My fingernails:
- A. Are manicured once in a while.

I just got married, and I got a beautiful ring with 12.5 little diamonds on it, so of course I have my nails done weekly.

- B. Are kept short and neat for simplicity.
- (C.) I have done weekly.

16. When it comes to athletics:
- A. Weekends are the only time I have for recreational sports.
- (B.) I'd only be more active if I were training for the Olympics.
- C. I hate to sweat.

Three times a week, Wednesday and Friday from 4:00 to 5:00 P.M. in the privacy of my home, thank you, I have an exercise splinner lesson.

17. If I have a little extra money to splurge with, I:
- A. Buy something I need.
- (B.) Get something for the kids.
- C. Buy something wonderful I've been dying to be tempted.

I'm all three. Let's have something for every one!

18. My idea of the perfect vacation would be to:
- (A.) Travel to the major cities of Europe.
- B. Go hiking and backpacking.
- C. Escape to a spa.

why limit it? money? Honey? to Europe? How about the whole world?

19. My bedtime is:
- (A.) After the 11:00 P.M. news.
- B. Early. After an exhausting day.
- C. Whenever the party's over.

Well, I've been to do all three, but I know the basically it's A.

20. If I could sum up my beauty routine simply, I would say it's:
- A. Sensible.
- (B.) Practical.
- C. Time-consuming.

what's the difference between sensible and practical? why don't you have "simple" on this test? well, it's practical to be simple, so there.

Jose says:

Brenda needs fullness on top, to make her face look narrower, and she looks wonderful with lots of hair. It's permed to give her a wild mane, and cut in long layers with lots of short hair framing the face so the length isn't dragged down. The short layers lift her hair at the sides. She can set her hair on small electric rollers in the morning and brush it out upside down to last all day. Brenda's hair looks like it is all one length, but it isn't and that is what makes the hairstyle work for her.

Barbara Walters

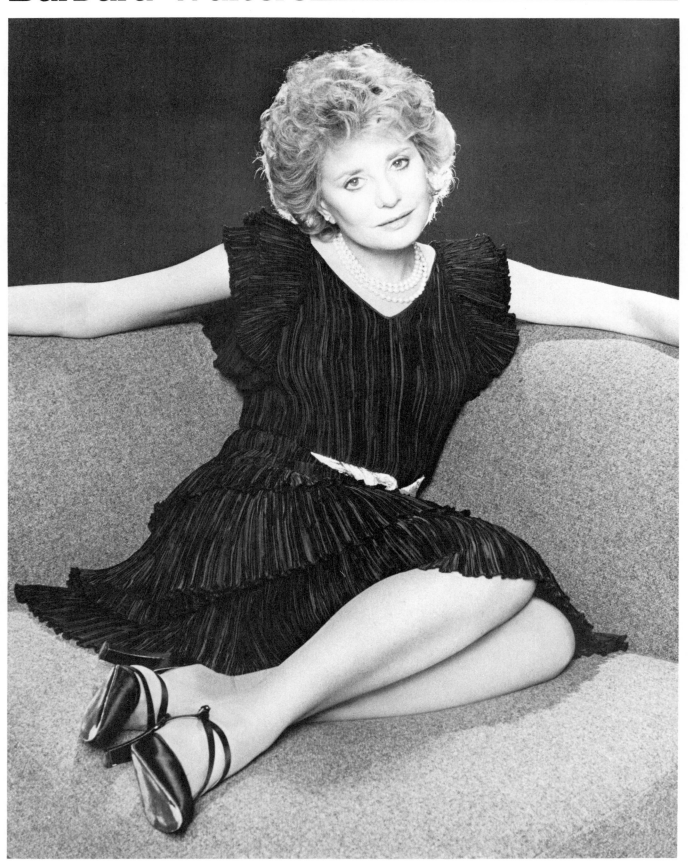

Barbara Walters is one of my most exciting clients, because every time I work with her, it is like being in the background of history. I go with her a lot of the time when she tapes her interviews, and I fix her hair, and then I stand next to the cameramen and the crew and I make sure her hair is right, so I get to be part of her incredible interviews. Through her I've met Katharine Hepburn, Paul Newman, Lauren Bacall, Clint Eastwood, Burt Reynolds, Walter Matthau—all kinds of famous people. We went to Patty Hearst's house; that was very nice. I went to the ranch in Santa Barbara when Barbara interviewed President Reagan, and I met the President and Mrs. Reagan. Then I went to the White House with Barbara when she interviewed Mrs. Reagan. We have had some incredible experiences together over the last four years.

For the White House I was very nervous, because I usually dress so flamboyantly, and I had to wear a conservative suit and tie. The crew and Barbara were all teasing me; they couldn't believe the way I was dressed. The visit to the ranch was less formal, so I could dress more casually. It was very strange to stand there and be eyed by so many security guards while I was doing Barbara's hair. The wind was blowing, and it was a very hard situation, but very exciting.

Right before the interview with Katharine Hepburn, after I had done Barbara's hair, Miss Hepburn asked if there was someone who could take care of her hair. The crew said, "Yes, sure, Jose is here." So she asked me what to do about her hair. I was speechless. When Katharine Hepburn asks you about her hair, what do you say? It wasn't as if she'd come into the shop and I could play around with it. So I just said that I thought it looked fine, and it did.

Working with Barbara has given me the opportunity to meet fascinating people and to go to places that most of us never can or do. It has been one of the most fabulous things in my life.

From my experience with Barbara, I'd say that, if she took my Life-style Quiz, she would be a Life-style Green. She's a very busy, very professional woman who, unless she is going in front of the camera, doesn't have too much time to spend on her hair or makeup. When I don't do her hair she usually washes and sets it herself in the morning before she leaves the house.

Barbara Walters' makeup by Tommy Cole.

Lesley Ann Warren

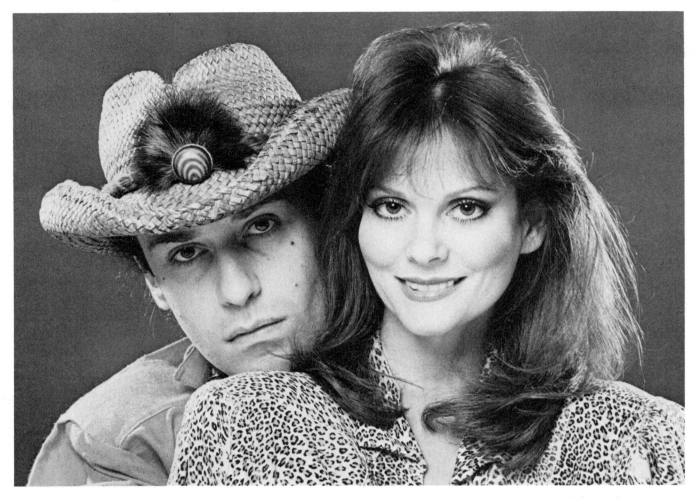

I had heard about Jose for years, ever since he first came to Beverly Hills. I had friends who went to him and I'd read about him, but I was really intimidated by who he was. He seemed like such a star, and I thought he'd be very snobbish, because his clientele was so exclusive. I felt too overwhelmed by all that to go to him. Then I ran into him at a benefit where I was modeling, and he was doing Cher's hair, and I found him really fascinating. So I made an appointment with him, but then I chickened out and canceled it. Finally I got up enough courage to go, but made my boyfriend come with me.

Well, Jose couldn't have been nicer. He was the opposite of everything I'd imagined. We've become fast friends, and we confide in each other, and we go out socially together.

Having been married to a hairdresser, I've had my hair violently changed according to his whims, and I didn't want to go to another person who would just do my hair his way and not listen to me. Jose and I pretty much agree about who I am, and we discuss each haircut in terms of my life as an actress and my personal life.

The first time I went to Jose, my hair was permed and growing out—it was between lengths—and it had no style. Jose gave me his famous tousled hairstyle, with semilayers and bangs, and it was perfect. I was going on location for a film in New Zealand, where I'd be outdoors, in the wind and near the ocean, and we had to work with those variables. Jose did it.

Basically we try to stick to simple, classic haircuts. We both prefer that my face come through the hairstyle. Now my hair is long, and I'm loving it. I use shampoo from a health-food store that gives it a great shine. I'm so health-oriented, I take a lot of vitamins and I exercise a lot, and that affects your hair. I can't stand for hair to look damaged. I'd rather have healthy hair than stylish hair, if it ever came to that, which of course it doesn't.

JOSE EBER'S LIFE-STYLE QUIZ   *Lesley Ann Warren*

1. **When I wake up in the morning:**
   - A. I look at the alarm clock and panic. I'm already late.
   - B. Who needs an alarm clock? I'm up with the birds, or the kids, and ready to go.
   - C. I roll over and go back to sleep for another half hour because last night really was a bit too much.

2. **My regular morning routine:**
   - A. Takes no more than half an hour because I'm so busy.
   - B. Is postponed until later in the day, because I'm out the door for tennis or carpool.
   - C. Depends on what I'm doing during the day and what's cooking for the upcoming evening.

3. **When I look in the mirror each morning I:**
   - A. Wish I had time to do something about what I see.
   - B. Splash cold water on my face and check the condition of my skin.
   - C. Study each line, blemish, and soft spot mercilessly, until I'm satisfied I know exactly how to best care for what I've seen.

4. **First thing in the morning, my hair:**
   - A. Needs a wash and blow-dry.
   - B. Kind of falls into place, because my haircut is easy to care for.
   - C. Is almost perfect, because I just had it done yesterday.

5. **My hair:**
   - A. Gets cut whenever I'm in the mood or can't do a thing with it.
   - B. Needs to be cut every four–six weeks; otherwise it's unmanageable.
   - C. Is long to allow me to manage a variety of hairstyles depending on my needs so I just make sure the ends are trimmed frequently.

6. **My hair color:**
   - A. Is something I've experimented with myself.
   - B. Yuck! Ruin my hair with chemicals?
   - C. Is done at the beauty shop every six weeks.

   Hmm, doesn't apply. It's A or C. I guess C.

7. **The colors I wear most frequently are:**
   - A. Neutrals that mix well in the business world: navy, burgundy, cream, and things that are "safe."
   - B. Bright colors, I love 'em.
   - C. Whatever the fashion mavens say is "in," as long as it's also flattering to my skin tones.

   I wear all colors

8. **For a purse, I usually carry:**
   - A. One good all-purpose bag that goes with all my clothes.
   - B. Something fun and inexpensive that holds all the junk I carry around.
   - C. Whatever matches my clothes.

9. **The hair appliances I rely on include:**
   - A. A round brush and blow-dryer.
   - B. I have all kinds of stuff, but I never use it.
   - C. Electric rollers, hairpins, combs, clips, curling iron, crimper, dryers, and brushes.

145

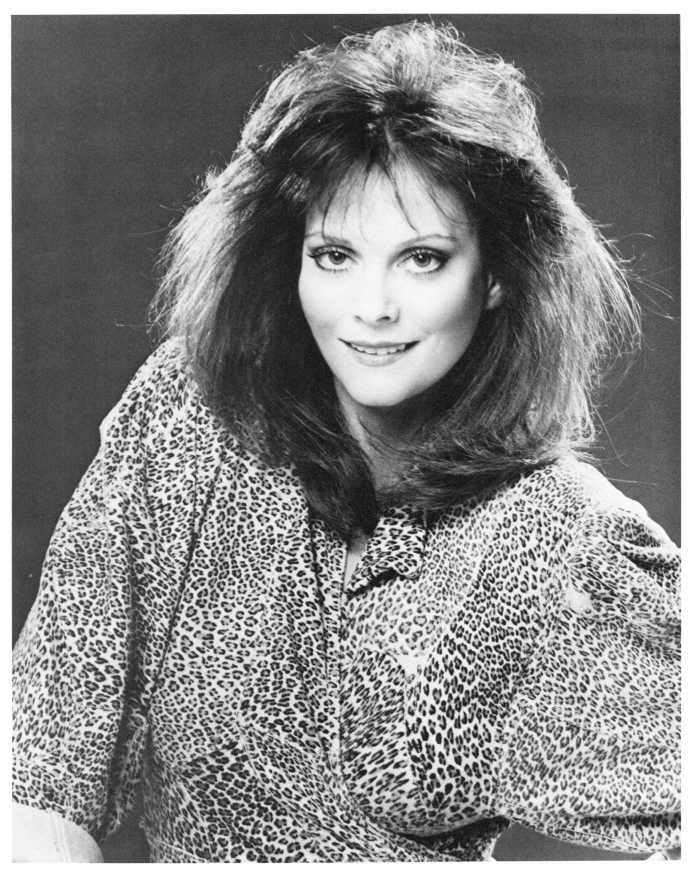

10. **For breakfast, I:**
    A. Grab something on the way to work or eat at my desk
    B. Have cold cereal and fruit.
    C. Eat a light meal if I'm dieting or a little more if I'm ~~having a late~~ lunch.

    I don't eat breakfast

11. **When I bathe, I:**
    A. Take a shower first thing in the morning.
    B. Take a shower several times a day, after tennis or swimming.
    C. Take a leisurely bath.

12. **I have help in my home:**
    A. Never.
    B. Once or twice a week.
    C. Full time.

13. **I put myself together:**
    A. To please myself.
    B. To suit my life-style.
    C. To please my man.

14. **I work:**
    A. Nine to five at a regular job.
    B. You think taking care of the kids isn't full-time work?
    C. Flexible hours or not at all.

15. **My fingernails:**
    A. Are manicured by me.

    B. Are kept short and neat for simplicity.
    C. I have done weekly.

16. **When it comes to athletics:**
    A. Weekends are the only time I have for recreational sports.
    B. I'd only be more active if I were training for the Olympics.
    C. I don't sweat.

17. **If I have a little extra money to splurge with, I:**
    A. Buy something I need.
    B. Get something for the kids.
    C. Buy something wonderful I've been dying to have.

18. **My idea of the perfect vacation would be to:**
    A. Travel to the major cities of Europe.
    B. Go hiking and backpacking.
    C. Escape to a spa.

19. **My bedtime is:**
    A. After the 11:00 P.M. news.
    B. Early, after an exhausting day.
    C. Whenever the party's over.

20. **If I could sum up my beauty routine simply, I would say it's:**
    A. Sensible.
    B. Practical.
    C. Time-consuming.

Jose says:
Lesley has such a small face that she cannot wear long bangs, so she likes the kind that are cut to the side. The rest of her hair is one length, with no layers and she doesn't have a perm. There are enough short pieces from the bangs for her to have a lot of versatility, and the pieces are long enough to be combed back, so she doesn't have to have bangs if she doesn't want them. Her eyes are huge and incredible, and we have to be careful that her face isn't hidden.

Life-style Blue.

PROFILE

When some women take my Life-style Quiz, they are embarrassed if they test Life-style Blue. They think this means they are lazy or that they have no purpose in life. They sometimes think it is better to test Red or Green.

Darling, this is all wrong. None of the three categories is better than the next. They are merely measurements of how much time you have to spend on your beauty look. If you are Life-style Blue, I say, be proud. Every woman is envious of you, believe me.

The women who get embarrassed are usually the ones who read magazine articles about young supermoms and feel they should be doing more. I think this is silly. What you need instead is to take stock of what you do and enjoy what you are able to achieve. Don't sell yourself short. How you look is probably important not only to you, but to your husband and your husband's line of work. Most Life-style Blues are professional wives, and this is a full-time job. So don't shrug it off too easily!

One of the things I like best about Life-style Blue women is that they truly appreciate style. Many tear pictures from magazines to show me styles they are considering. Others may bring in a blouse or a dress and ask me to create a hairstyle to fit the mood of the garment for a special occasion. The few Life-style Blues I encounter who aren't stunning are stuck in what I call a Blue Rut. They don't realize that they could look ten years younger. They don't know how to achieve the right style, which they could handle themselves and still look very elegant and classy.

Many times a Life-style Blue lives in a small city and cannot get the kind of haircut she deserves. Or else, no matter where she lives, she has been going to the same hairdresser for fifteen years and hasn't changed her hairstyle in that long. That's part of the Blue Rut syndrome. She doesn't know she's in it; she's embarrassed to change hairstylists because she is so loyal or she doesn't want to hurt anyone's feelings. She may also be nervous about making a change—after all, in fifteen years she has gotten used to whatever she's been doing so regularly.

So the trick is to escape Blue Rut without being blue. Don't be nervous and don't be shy. Pay special attention to the women in this life-style section and bring this book to your hairdresser. Don't suggest that he imitate someone else's look for you—that will never do! Do suggest that together you go over your worksheet and examine the Life-style Blue hairstyles so you can find one that fits your face and your life-style variables. Time is on the side of the Life-style Blue woman—she can experiment and work with a stylist. She should take advantage of her good fortune.

Once the Life-style Blue woman has the right haircut, she has the time to arrange her hair in any number of styles. She uses electric rollers almost every day, or possibly daily. She also uses a hair dryer and curling iron, and may use rollers or curling papers for a different type of set.

Because the Blue lady does not go to work in the morning, her schedule is more relaxed. She probably has time to eat breakfast and read the paper or watch a television talk show or news program. She may do charity work or make phone calls to friends. She may exercise to a tape or record. She may even sleep late. She knows the importance of sleep for her good looks, so she's careful to catch up in the morning with what she may have missed the night before.

For a woman in this category, the days are usually different. She has family and social obligations and makes appearances with her husband, as well as doing charity work and errands and lunching with friends. If she has several functions in one day, the Life-style Blue woman may come home to change her clothes and rearrange her hair. She spends a lot of time on self-presentation, and likes to make sure she is perfect whenever she goes out in public. This is a woman who watches her weight, is usually on a diet, and is very careful about the kind and amount of food she eats. She checks her skin for signs of age, uses whatever new beauty products and skin creams are on the market, and has her nails done regularly. Her choice of a vacation spot would be a spa, where she can get away from the pressures of being perfect.

Life-style Blues are not strangers to beauty salons, and many have a standing weekly appointment. They usually have their hair color done professionally, and rarely perform any beauty tasks on themselves or their friends. They are willing to pay to have a service performed so it comes out perfectly. They don't like to mess around with do-it-yourself products unless they are guaranteed satisfaction.

Older Life-style Blues may be uncomfortable using a hand-held dryer and electric rollers, because they are used to total salon care. If this sounds familiar, you could well be suffering from Blue Rut. If you had a style you loved, which you could do yourself, wouldn't you be happier?

Life-style Blues have hair of all lengths. Most of my Life-style Blue women have longish hair, because it's so versatile. But I've met many Blues who think that as they age they must keep their hair shorter and shorter. This is a matter of choice, and should be just one of the other variables in their lives. Believe me, age should not dictate your hair length; if any life-style is perfect for long hair, it is Blue.

I'm not saying that if you have short hair you should let it grow immediately, darling. But the beauty of being Life-style Blue is that you have more choices than anyone else, so don't eliminate long hair as a possibility.

Since Life-style Blues don't work, it is safe to assume that they have no severe financial problems. Often Life-style Blues are a little more flush than other women. They can afford to get all their beauty services performed professionally. Life-style

Blues don't usually have to save for something they need, and they tend to splurge on luxuries or extravagances for themselves or friends and loved ones.

Because their time is their own, Life-style Blues often prefer a bath to a shower. Many shower in the morning (and wash their hair) and then take a relaxing bath in the late afternoon or early evening. They may have full-time help; they seldom have small children at home.

Life-style Blues are very conscious of wearing an outfit that's right for the situation. They change their handbag to match their clothes. They shop with their husband or get their husband's approval on their purchases. The Life-style Blue woman's personal look is often defined by her husband.

Life-style Blues are not big on sporting activities. Because looking good is important to them, they exercise, not because they like to, but because they think they have to. They seldom go in for group sports but may not mind watching them. They are concerned with keeping their bodies trim but are not the type to play tennis all day, jog in the morning, or meet their husband for a quick, passionate game of racquetball after work.

Life-style Blue women are usually very good with makeup and know full well that the right kind adds the finishing touch to a hairstyle. Sometimes I have to remind a Life-style Blue woman not to overdo the makeup, but this is rare.

Life-style Blues are usually social creatures. They like to party, and enjoy social obligations tied in with their husband's position. If they don't like to entertain at home, it's not unusual for them to take friends to a nice restaurant. Life-style Blues go to cocktail parties and charity balls at least a few times a year. Their husband or boyfriend may complain about wearing a tuxedo, but Blue ladies like to dress up. Invariably they go to a stylist to create a special style for these big occasions.

The Blue woman has time to change her clothes, redo her hairstyle, and make sure that everything about her look is perfect before she goes out at night. Celebrities often test Life-style Blue because it's their business to look beautiful. Deep in their heart, they may have other ideas, but because they can't go out in public looking anything less than gorgeous, they have to spend more time on their looks than they would generally.

HOW TO SHAMPOO YOUR HAIR

Although you go to the beauty salon more often than other women, you still need to wash your hair at home. Some Life-style Blues like to have the kind of hairstyle that comes from the beauty salon and sits on their head without moving for several days. Then, when the style begins to fade, they go back to the salon for a comb-out or reluctantly wash their hair. I think this is old-fashioned. It's just the "done" look I am fighting. I want my Life-style Blues to be able to do their own hair and to have a soft, natural, crushable look. So throw out your hair spray, Ms. Blue, and wash your hair each morning or every other morning.

150

Have several varieties of mild shampoo on hand and alternate often. Use a lot of water and make sure your hair is very wet before you apply the shampoo. If you have long hair, spend a minute or two getting your hair totally wet. Use the shampoo and massage your scalp while washing your hair—don't forget the hairline as well. Rinse carefully with plenty of water and then use creme rinse. You do not need more than one shampooing. Chances are, your hair takes as much abuse as the Life-style Red woman's, so make sure you are using a very mild shampoo.

CONDITIONING

Blue women may prefer to have their deep conditioning done in the salon. But when they wash their hair (or have it washed in the salon), creme rinse should be used, especially on the ends, which have a tendency to dry out from the constant use of electric rollers. For this reason, trimming is important too.

The Life-style Blue has the time to condition her hair properly and does not need to worry about doing a quickie foil wrap while watching television or helping the kids with their homework. Nor need she worry about her husband's teasing while she walks around the house with mayonnaise in her hair, wearing a big turban. She can do all her conditioning while her husband is at work, on her own time schedule. One of the best ways for a Blue woman to condition is in the morning, when she's on her own. She can put on deep conditioner, wrap her hair in a towel or aluminum foil, and sit under a hood-style dryer for maximum heat conditioning. If she doesn't want to use the hair dryer, she can talk on the telephone and make her morning calls or do her correspondence while all wrapped up. Then she can shower and wash her hair (there's no need for creme rinse now) and proceed with her regular morning styling.

HOW TO DRY YOUR HAIR

Because there are so many possibilities for damaging their hair, Life-style Blues have to be extremely careful with their hair drying. It is very bad to overdry your hair with a blow-dryer and to then use electric rollers every day! If you can let your hair dry naturally—you may even want to wrap it—it is better for you. Wrapping is a very American technique and is popular with people who don't have a lot of time to straighten their hair or even to set it with rollers, but who don't want to let their hair dry naturally for fear it will kink and curl too much and be very wild and have no shape. When you hair wrap, you are giving your hair just enough curl because the curl comes from the curves of your head!

Hair wrapping is for long hair only! If your hair is not long enough to go around your head at least once, don't even try this method.

Your hair must be wet in order to wrap it properly. So:

1. Wash or spritz hair till totally wet.
2. Apply setting lotion if you want a little extra oomph and body. Setting lotion will also help straighten naturally curly hair.
3. Comb through your hair carefully.
4. Make a part on the left or right crown.
5. Moving in the direction of the part, wrap the hair against the head as tightly as possible. Clip it with those long skinny metal clips to hold flat. Do not use the little clips, as they will leave marks.
6. Pull and stretch your hair as you wrap it around, making sure it lies smoothly. Bumps and squiggles will show up when the hair dries.
7. Wrap completely around the head as many times as your hair goes.
8. Let dry. Unpin. Comb out. (Do not sleep on wrapped hair.)

Then you won't need to worry about burning or heat damage. An infrared lamp is something else you should consider, or an old-fashioned hood dryer. If you use a blow-dryer, it should be to take moisture out, not to style your hair. Electric rollers will take care of the styling later on.

If you are one of the few Life-style Blues who is good with a blow-dryer, congratulations. You may be able to style your hair yourself with a round brush and the dryer, and just use rollers or a curling iron for light curling. But if you use electric rollers everyday, like most Life-style Blues, beware of overdrying.

PERMANENTS

A permanent wave is not a necessity for a Life-style Blue lady, because she is already using her electric rollers every day and is checking her hair whenever she goes out. If the hair is baby-fine or stick-straight, then a light perm should be considered. The hair condition has to be maintained, because if you have colored hair and you use electric rollers regularly, you must be very careful that you don't damage your hair with chemicals. Be sure that your perm is done at the salon, by a professional. This is not something for you to attempt at home!

COLORING

Since most Life-style Blues are over forty, they usually have colored hair to cover up the gray. This is nice, because gray hair usually makes you look older. I have seen many stunning women with gray hair, but it is probably not right for you.

Life-style Blues should have their hair color done professionally, at a salon, although sometimes they like to do the simple color processes themselves. Color should always be kept natural, perhaps a touch lighter than the natural shade, but never darker—this makes a woman look old or hard.

TO SPRAY OR NOT TO SPRAY

There is absolutely no reason why a Life-style Blue woman should use hair spray. It's very old-fashioned, and I hate it. The lacquered look is dead, darling. And your hair does not need one more thing that might damage its condition! If you feel the need to spray your hair to keep it in place, you have the wrong hairstyle and the wrong haircut. With all the advantages you have as a Life-style Blue, you can always look fresh, soft, sexy, and dynamic, totally without hair spray.

SUPPLIES

Daily
electric rollers

Every other day or frequently
mild shampoo
blow-dryer
creme rinse
curling iron
deep conditioner

Occasionally
tissue paper and bobby pins
hairpins
crimper
combs
ribbons, headbands, assorted fashion
　accessories
old-fashioned (nonelectric) rollers
hood-style hair dryer
infrared light blubs for drying

YOUR MORNING SCHEDULE

- 8:00–9:00 A.M.: Wake up
- Have breakfast (or coffee)while watching television news or talk show, reading newspaper
- Go over mail: 20–30 minutes
- Shower and wash hair: 20 minutes or bathe (no shampoo): 15 minutes

- Hairstyling: 30 minutes
- Make up: 15–20 minutes
- Dress: 15 minutes

- Total beauty routine: 60 minutes*
- Total morning routine: 2 hours*

*does not include exercising or deep conditioning

Barbara Carrera

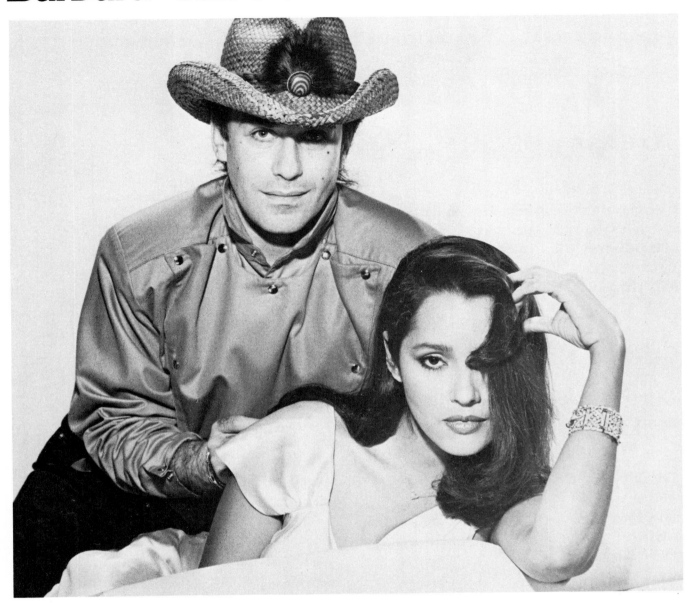

I went to Jose because I wanted him to get rid of Clay Baskets for me. I played Clay Baskets, an Indian woman, in a television epic, "Centennial," and the shooting was very long and hard. Clay Baskets had to age over a period of years, and I'd had it up to my ears with the whole thing. I wanted to shave my armpits and cut off my hair and get a new look. I just said to Jose, "Cut." He did, to my shoulders, and I started wearing my hair to one side, and since then he's been taking care of it.

Last summer he cut it much too short, but it was my fault. We were having a photo session, he was late, and I was looking through magazines and saw a picture that I showed to him, and that was that. I'm impetuous, and unfortunately Jose is too, so before we knew it, the hair was off. It was too short. But then, a little later, I had to wear a wig for a film I was making in which the character was a Russian woman with dark-blond hair. My hair is too dark to color blond, so I had to wear a wig, and since my hair was so short, it worked out all right. It was fun to have short hair for about a month. But I got it out of my system.

I don't pick a hairstyle based on too many variables; it depends mostly on what's the right look for me. And I don't like too much hair, which makes my face look round. When the hair's away from the face, I look better.

JOSE EBER'S LIFE-STYLE QUIZ

Barbara Carrera (handwritten)

1. When I wake up in the morning, have any
   A. I wake up late. I look at the alarm clock and panic. I'm already late.
   B. Who needs an alarm clock? I'm up with the birds or the kids, and ready to go.
   C. I roll over and go back to sleep for another half hour because last night really was a bit too much.

(handwritten) It's B and C. In New York I look at the alarm clock and panic. In Paris California, I'm a true birds out I don't go time limit so I'm working C, I guess I'm working with the birds or the kids

2. **My regular morning routine:**
   A. Takes no more than half an hour because I'm so busy.
   B. Is postponed until later in the day, because I'm out the door for tennis or carpool.
   C. Depends on what I'm doing during the day and what's cooking for the upcoming evening.

3. **When I look in the mirror each morning I:**
   A. Wish I had time to do something about what I see.
   B. Splash cold water on my face and check the condition of my skin.
   C. Study each line, blemish, and soft spot mercilessly until I'm satisfied I know exactly how to best care for what I've seen.

(handwritten) I only look in the mirror when I brush my teeth.

4. **First thing in the morning, my hair:**
   A. Needs a wash and blow-dry.
   B. Kind of falls into place, because my hair's easy to care for.
   C. Is almost perfect because I washed it yesterday.

(handwritten) It's A or B. I don't have a routine. Either I wash it because it's going out or it kind of falls into place. It depends on whether it needs to be washed.

5. **My hair:**
   A. Gets cut whenever I'm in the mood or can't do a thing with it.
   B. Needs to be cut every four–six weeks; otherwise it's unmanageable.
   C. Is long to allow me to manage a variety of hairstyles depending on my needs so I just make sure the ends are trimmed frequently.

6. **My hair color:**
   A. Is something I've experimented with myself.
   B. Yuck my hair with chemicals? It's done at the beauty shop every six weeks.
   C.

(handwritten) I don't play with my hair color regularly. But I like to experiment when I'm in the mood

7. **The colors I wear most frequently are:**
   A. Neutrals that mix well in the business world: navy, burgundy, cream, and things that are safe.
   B. Bright colors. I love 'em.
   C. Whatever the fashion mavens say is "in," as long as it's also flattering to skin tones.

(handwritten) It's not A. Really I like black, and it's not C. white for summer and red for winter and black for winter between.

8. **For a purse, I usually carry:**
   A. One good all-purpose bag that goes with all my clothes.
   B. Something fun and inexpensive that holds all the junk I carry around.
   C. Whatever matches my clothes.

(handwritten) It's always A. I change pain handbags.

9. **The hair appliances I rely on include:**
   A. A round brush and blow-dryer.
   B. I have all kinds of stuff, but I never use it.
   C. Electric rollers, hairpins, combs, clips, curling iron, crimper, dryers, and brushes.

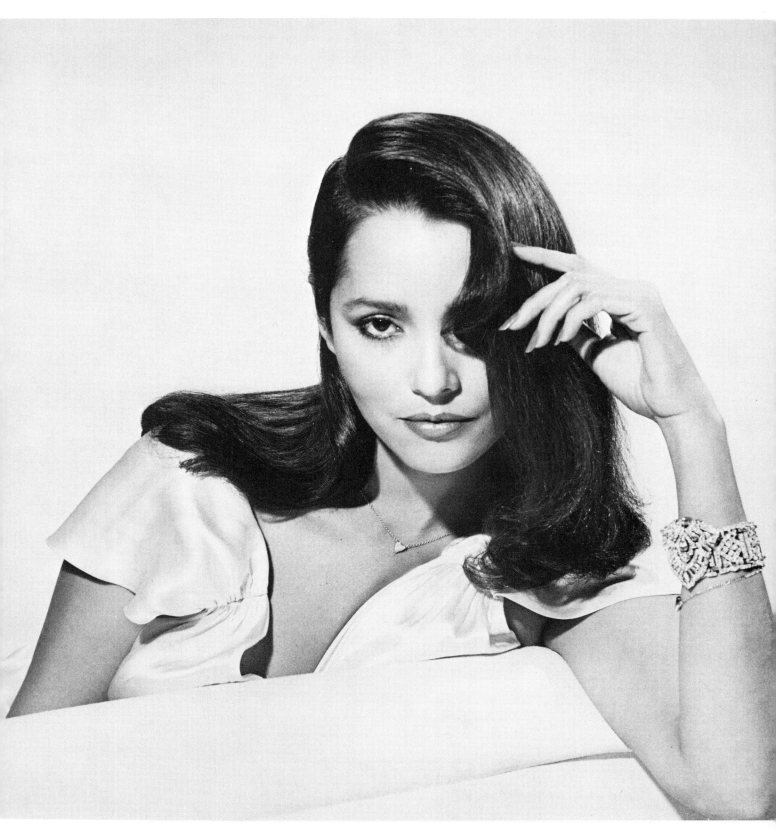

10. **For breakfast, I:**
    A. Grab something on the way to work or eat at my desk.
    B. Have cold cereal and fruit.
    C. Eat a light meal if I'm dieting or a little more if I'm having a late lunch.

I don't usually eat but when I do, a real breakfast. I do, a real feast.

11. **When I bathe, I:**
    A. Take a shower first thing in the morning.
    B. Take a shower several times a day, after tennis or swimming.
    (C). Take a leisurely bath.

I love baths!

12. **I have help in my home:**
    A. Never.
    B. Once or twice a week.
    (C). Full time.

These questions are so funny.

13. **I put myself together:**
    (A) To please myself.
    B. To suit my life-style.
    C. To please my partner.

I dress to suit my mood. If I'm with a lover, I dress to please him. There are exceptions to the rules.

14. **I work:**
    A. Nine to five at a regular job.
    B. You think taking care of the kids isn't full-time work?
    C. Flexible hours or not at all.

15. **My fingernails:**
    A. Are manicured by me.
    (B) Are kept short and neat for simplicity.
    C. I have done weekly.

I play the guitar so I keep them short.

16. **When it comes to athletics:**
    A. Weekends are the only time I have for recreational sports.
    (B) I'd only be more active if I were training for the Olympics.
    C. A sport or exercise is a way of life for me. I have almost a complete gym at my home.

my house   *I don't sweat*

17. **If I have a little extra money to splurge with I:**
    A. Buy something I need for every day.
    B. Get something for the kids.
    C. Buy some champagne.

It depends on my mood today. I'm feeling generous, for every body's parties for the crew. But if I had a lot of extra money then I'd buy a house.

18. **My idea of the perfect vacation would be to:**
    A. Travel to the major cities of Europe.
    B. Go hiking and backpacking.
    (C) Escape to a spa.

Do I have to choose? To me the most definitely the perfect holiday is to get away from every body, and if there are people at the spa, forget it. I'll take a primitive island near the Seychelles!

19. **My bedtime is:**
    A. After the 11:00 P.M. news.
    B. Early, after an exhausting day.
    (C) Whenever the party's over.

It's a little... all three I guess.

20. **If I could sum up my beauty routine simply, I would say it's:**
    (A) Sensible.
    B. Practical.
    C. Time-consuming.

In this society, appearances count, and it's sensible to have good looks, otherwise I'd eat myself fat!

Jose says:
Barbara has such a stunning face, she can wear her hair any way, but the one I like best for her is when it's one length, long, so we can fool around with it and make her look different. We do this by keeping all the hair off her face. She can even wear it all pulled back at the nape of her neck. She has no perm, she lets her hair dry naturally, and she doesn't need any fullness, so we can just play and do whatever style she feels like.

Joanna Carson

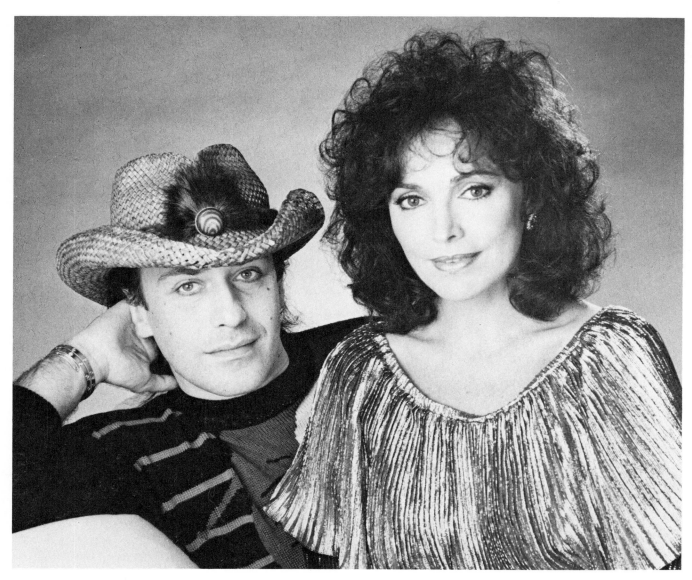

Joanna Carson is a working woman and the wife of a very important man—Johnny Carson. Since she is vice-president of Michaele Vollbracht Design, Inc., she is in the fashion world. And as Johnny's wife she is always in the spotlight. Although Joanna is one of the few women who look beautiful without makeup, she needs to take time with her hair and face to make sure she looks perfect when she steps out in public.

Her morning routine is devoted to telephone work—she must get up very early in Los Angeles to call New York in the morning. She usually concentrates on her business until lunchtime, eats a light lunch, and then does charity work until three-thirty or four o'clock in the afternoon. She is very active in several charities and is president of SHARE, a local organization. From four o'clock until six-thirty Joanna has what she calls her "wind-down time"—so she relaxes, takes a bath, and fixes her hair and makeup before Johnny comes home from the studio. When her husband gets home, they eat dinner and usually have a quiet evening at home.

Joanna is very careful about the condition of her hair and has it treated in New York by Dr. Philip Kingsley. She also uses his hair products. She started coming to me a little over a year ago, when she met a friend from Texas in a hotel lobby in Paris and began to talk about California hairdressers! I like to give her a style that is soft and sexy and full but still very natural-looking.

JOSE EBER'S LIFE-STYLE QUIZ

Joanna Carson

1. **When I wake up in the morning:**
   A. I look at the alarm clock and panic. I'm already late.
   B. Who needs an alarm clock? I'm up with the birds, or the kids, and ready to go.
   C. I roll over and go back to sleep for another half hour because last night really was a bit too much.

   D. when I wake up and I'm happy & hungry.

2. **My regular morning routine:**
   A. Takes no more than half an hour because I'm so busy.
   B. Is postponed until later in the day, because I'm out the door for tennis or carpool.
   C. Depends on what I'm doing during the day and what's cooking for the upcoming evening.

3. **When I look in the mirror each morning I:**
   A. Wish I had time to do something about what I see.
   B. Splash cold water on my face and check the condition of my skin.
   C. Study each line, blemish, and soft spot mercilessly, until I'm satisfied I know exactly how to best care for what I've seen.

   I splash a lot of water on my face.

4. **First thing in the morning, my hair:**
   A. Needs a wash and blow-dry.
   B. Kind of falls into place, because my haircut is easy to care for.
   C. Is almost perfect, because I just had it done yesterday.

5. **My hair:**
   A. Gets cut whenever I'm in the mood or can't do a thing with it.
   B. Needs to be cut every four–six weeks; otherwise it's unmanageable.
   C. Is long to allow me to manage a variety of hairstyles depending on my needs so I just make sure the ends are trimmed frequently.

6. **My hair color:**
   A. Is something I've experimented with myself.
   B. Yuck! Ruin my hair with chemicals?
   C. Is done at my beauty shop every six weeks.

   I do nothing to my hair color maybe it should be but it's getting to be about that time

7. **The colors I wear most frequently are:**
   A. Neutrals that mix well in the business world: navy, burgundy, cream, and things that are "safe."
   B. Bright colors, I love 'em.
   C. Whatever the fashion mavens say is "in," as long as it's also flattering to my skin tones.

8. **For a purse, I usually carry:**
   A. One good all-purpose bag that goes with all my clothes.
   B. Something fun and inexpensive that holds all the junk I carry around.
   C. Whatever matches my clothes.

9. **The hair appliances I rely on include:**
   A. A round brush and blow-dryer.
   B. I have all kinds of stuff, but I never use it.
   C. Electric rollers, hairpins, combs, clips, curling iron, crimper, dryers, and brushes.

159

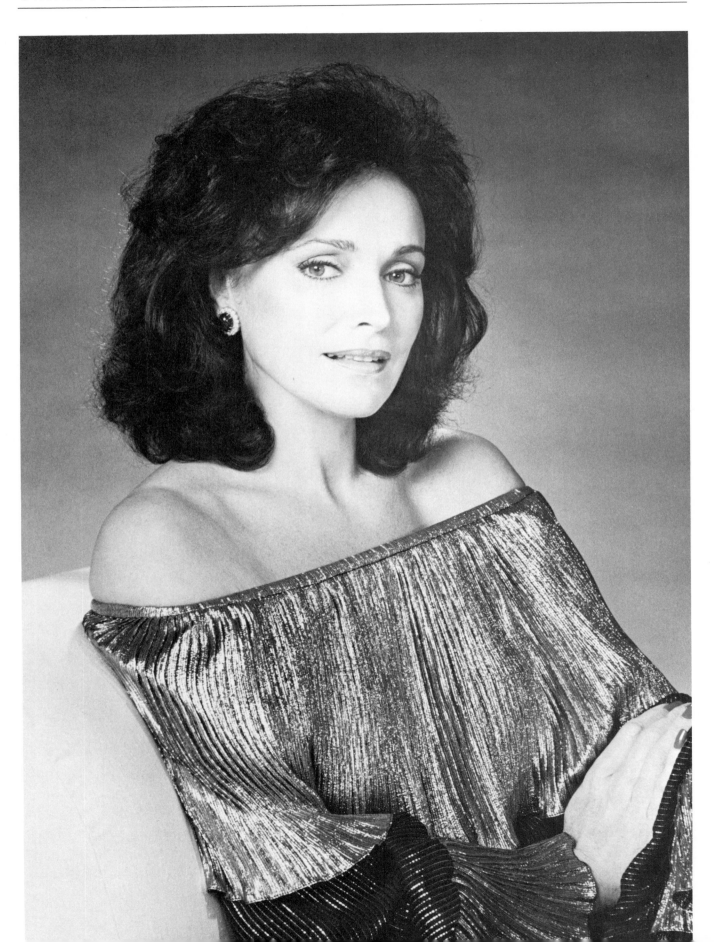

10. **For breakfast, I:**
    A. Grab something on the way to work or eat at my desk
    B. Have cold cereal and fruit.
    C. Eat a light meal if I'm dieting or a little more if I'm having a late lunch.

11. **When I bathe, I:**
    A. Take a shower first thing in the morning.
    B. Take a shower several times a day, after tennis or swimming.
    C. Take a leisurely bath.

12. **I have help in my home:**
    A. Never.
    B. Once or twice a week.
    C. Full time.

13. **I put myself together:**
    A. To please myself.
    B. To suit my life-style.
    C. To please my man.

14. **I work:**
    A. Nine to five at a regular job.
    B. You think taking care of the kids isn't full-time work?
    C. Flexible hours or not at all.

15. **My fingernails:**
    A. Are manicured by me.
    B. Are kept short and neat for simplicity.
    C. I have done weekly.

16. **When it comes to athletics:**
    A. Weekends are the only time I have for recreational sports.
    B. I'd only be more active if I were training for the Olympics.
    C. I don't sweat.

    I go to exercise class religiously three times a week.

17. **If I have a little extra money to splurge with, I:**
    A. Buy something I need.
    B. Get something for the kids.
    C. Buy something wonderful I've been dying to have.

18. **My idea of the perfect vacation would be to:**
    A. Travel to the major cities of Europe.
    B. Go hiking and backpacking.
    C. Escape to a spa.

19. **My bedtime is:**
    A. After the 11:00 P.M. news.
    B. Early, after an exhausting day.
    C. Whenever the party's over.

    D. After the monologue.

20. **If I could sum up my beauty routine simply, I would say it's:**
    A. Sensible.
    B. Practical.
    C. Time-consuming.

Jose says:
Being as glamorous as she is, and taking as good care of her hair as she does, Joanna can do just about anything with it. Thanks to her face shape, she can wear almost any style, and she has really curly hair, so she can let it dry naturally for a funky look, or use rollers for a more sophisticated one, or she can blow-dry it straight. This is a versatile cut, to suit whatever Joanna wants to do or look like. She has some different lengths cut on top, so she can wear bangs or pull all her hair back, away from the face.

Cher

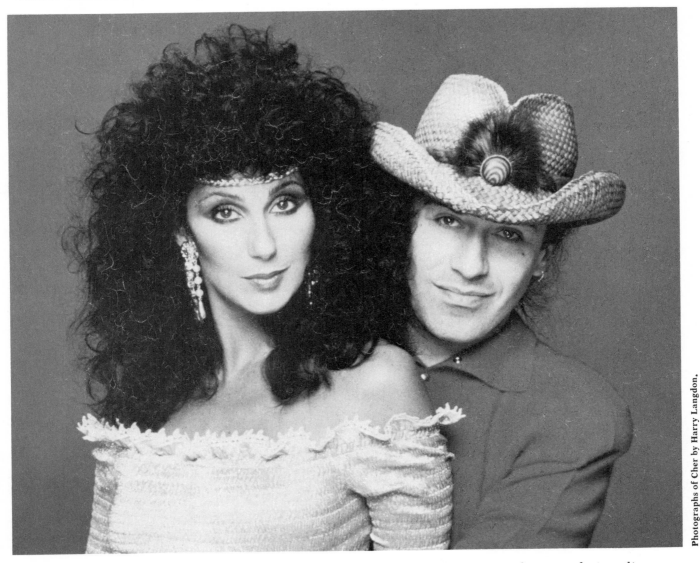

Photographs of Cher by Harry Langdon.

I heard from Susie Coehlo and Farrah and Kate Jackson that there was a hot new hairstylist in town. Also, Sonny had been having his lovely locks cut by him, and even Chastity was having him cut her hair, so I figured this was a family affair and I might as well get in on the act.

I had had my real really long hair cut when I was in London, so it reached about the middle of my back after the cut that was four and a half, maybe five, years ago. When I went to Jose, I trusted him right away. Then we did some photo sessions and TV specials together, and if I wanted my hair cut at one o'clock in the morning because that was the only time I had—since my schedule is so crazy—well, Jose came over and cut my hair. We're both night people. The time we cut my hair really short, it was midnight. It was a spontaneous decision. The next day, I decided to let it grow long again.

JOSE EBER'S LIFE-STYLE QUIZ *Cher*

1. **When I wake up in the morning:**
   A. I look at the alarm clock and panic. I'm already late.
   B. Who needs an alarm clock? I'm up with the birds, or the kids, and ready to go.
   C. I roll over and go back to sleep for another half hour because last night really was a bit too much.

   D. All of the above.

2. **My regular morning routine:**
   A. Takes no more than half an hour because I'm so busy.
   B. Is postponed until later in the day, because I'm out the door for tennis or carpool.
   C. Depends on what I'm doing during the day and what's cooking for the upcoming evening.

3. **When I look in the mirror each morning I:**
   A. Wish I had time to do something about what I see.
   B. Splash cold water on my face and check the condition of my skin.
   C. Study each line, blemish, and soft spot mercilessly, until I'm satisfied I know exactly how to best care for what I've seen.

4. **First thing in the morning, my hair:**
   A. Needs a wash and blow-dry.
   B. Kind of falls into place, because my haircut is easy to care for.
   C. Is almost perfect, because I just had it done yesterday.

5. **My hair:**
   A. Gets cut whenever I'm in the mood or can't do a thing with it.
   B. Needs to be cut every four–six weeks; otherwise it's unmanageable.
   C. Is long to allow me to manage a variety of hairstyles depending on my needs so I just make sure the ends are trimmed frequently.

6. **My hair color:**
   A. Is something I've experimented with myself.
   B. Yuck! Ruin my hair with chemicals?
   C. Is done at the beauty shop every six weeks.

7. **The colors I wear most frequently are:**
   A. Neutrals that mix well in the business world: navy, burgundy, cream, and things that are "safe."
   B. Bright colors, I love 'em.
   C. Whatever the fashion mavens say is "in," as long as it's also flattering to my skin tones.

8. **For a purse, I usually carry:**
   A. One good all-purpose bag that goes with all my clothes.
   B. Something fun and inexpensive that holds all the junk I carry around.
   C. Whatever matches my clothes.

9. **The hair appliances I rely on include:**
   A. A round brush and blow-dryer.
   B. I have all kinds of stuff, but I never use it.
   C. Electric rollers, hairpins, combs, clips, curling iron, crimper, dryers, and brushes.

   Depends.

163

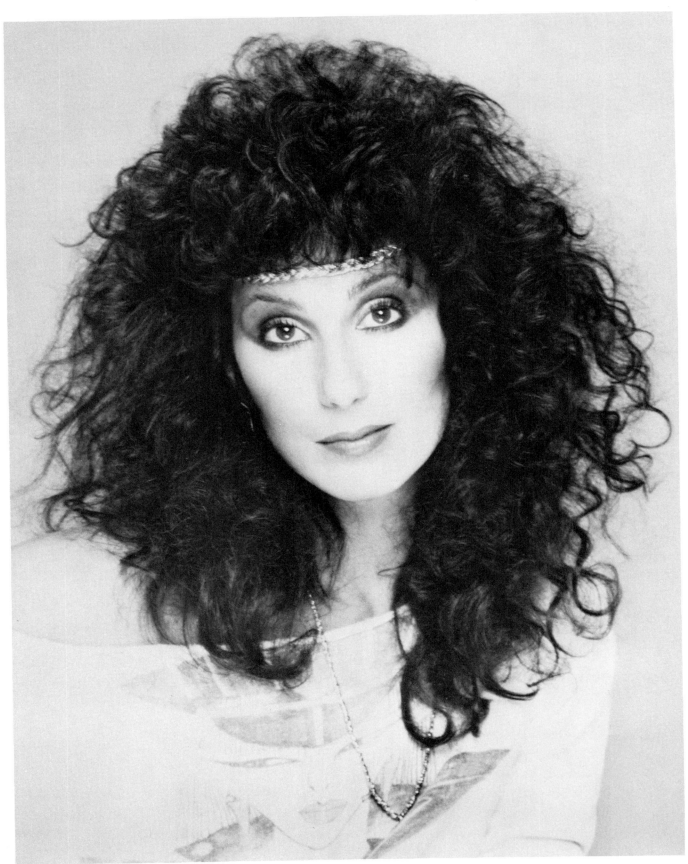

10. **For breakfast, I:**
    A. Grab something on the way to work or eat at my desk
    B. Have cold cereal and fruit.
    C. Eat a light meal if I'm dieting or a little more if I'm having a late lunch.

11. **When I bathe, I:**
    A. Take a shower first thing in the morning.
    B. Take a shower several times a day, after tennis or swimming.
    C. Take a leisurely bath.

12. **I have help in my home:**
    A. Never.
    B. Once or twice a week.
    C. Full time.

13. **I put myself together:**
    A. To please myself.
    B. To suit my life-style.
    C. To please my man.

14. **I work:**
    A. Nine to five at a regular job.
    B. You think taking care of the kids isn't full-time work?
    C. Flexible hours or not at all.

15. **My fingernails:**
    A. Are manicured by me.

B. Are kept short and neat for simplicity.
    C. I have done weekly.

16. **When it comes to athletics:**
    A. Weekends are the only time I have for recreational sports.
    B. I'd only be more active if I were training for the Olympics.
    C. I don't sweat.

17. **If I have a little extra money to splurge with, I:**
    A. Buy something I need.
    B. Get something for the kids.
    C. Buy something wonderful I've been dying to have.

18. **My idea of the perfect vacation would be to:**
    A. Travel to the major cities of Europe.
    B. Go hiking and backpacking.
    C. Escape to a spa.

19. **My bedtime is:**
    A. After the 11:00 P.M. news.
    B. Early, after an exhausting day.
    C. Whenever the party's over.

20. **If I could sum up my beauty routine simply, I would say it's:**
    A. Sensible.
    B. Practical.
    C. Time-consuming.

Darling this is drama!

Jose says:
Cher can wear anything. She feels more comfortable with long hair, but she has had short hair too. She has extremely straight hair and no perm. We get the volume she likes, and make curls by rolling with tissue paper. The top section of her hair is cut shorter than the rest so we can get volume and shape. Cher loves to look different constantly, and this haircut allows her to.

Angie Dickinson

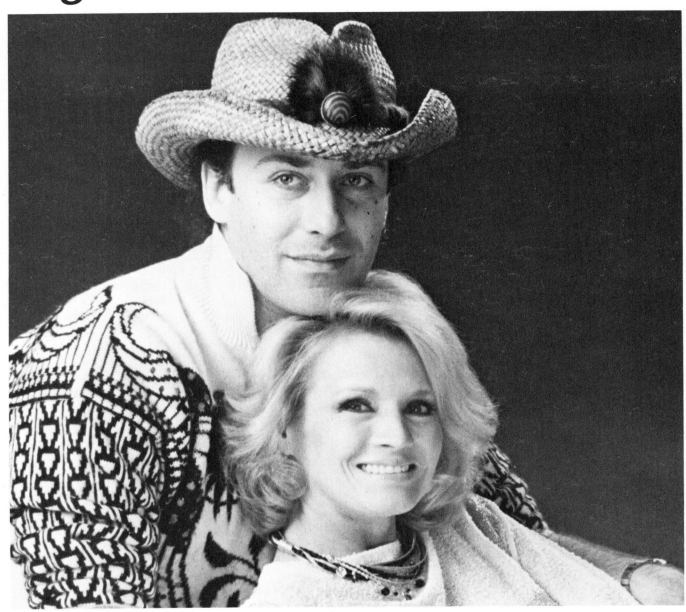

I first met Jose through my commercials agent, Marge Schicktanz. Marge goes to Jose (see page 130), and so do some of her other friends, and she kept telling me that she thought he would give my hair the little extra help it always needs. I have fine hair—it's baby-fine—and it needs just the right cut and style to stay in place. I figured I had nothing to lose, and Marge always looks great, so why not?

Well, Jose and I hit it off immediately. And ever since then, he's done my hair for special occasions—he's flown to New York with me for commercials; if I'm doing the "Tonight" show, he comes to the studio and fixes my hair beforehand; he works on it for awards or anything else. Jose is always there for me—he's worked on his day off, on Sundays, late at night. And when he does my hair, it lasts.

He gave me a perm on the roots—great idea, isn't it? And since my hair has always dropped, I can tell you that a root perm is really a miracle. It adds lots of body. The perm holds up my hair so it doesn't go flat, and I keep a good bit of length to get the fullness I need. We set my hair with electric curlers—just for a few seconds, because I don't want to damage my hair, which is very fragile, and Jose understands it. And that's all there is to it.

166

JOSE EBER'S LIFE-STYLE QUIZ

Angie Dickinson

1. When I wake up in the morning:
  A. I look at the alarm clock and panic. I'm already late.
  B. Who needs an alarm clock? I'm up with the birds, or the kids, and ready to go.
  C. I roll over and go back to sleep for another half hour because last night really was a bit too much.

2. My regular morning routine:
  A. Takes no more than half an hour because I'm so busy.
  B. Is postponed until later in the day, because I'm out the door for tennis or carpool.
  C. Depends on what I'm doing during the day and what's cooking for the upcoming evening.

3. When I look in the mirror each morning I:
  A. Wish I had time to do something about what I see.
  B. Splash cold water on my face and check the condition of my skin.
  C. Study each line, blemish, and soft spot mercilessly, until I'm satisfied I know exactly how to best care as what I've seen.

  D. I decide to put it off as long as possible.

4. First thing in the morning, my hair:
  A. Needs a wash and blow-dry.
  B. Kind of falls into place, because my haircut is easy to care for.
  C. Is almost perfect because I just had it done yesterday.

  D. also in the afternoon or evening if I'm going somewhere special.

5. My hair:
  A. Gets cut whenever I'm in the mood or can spare a thing to fix it.
  B. Needs to be cut every four–six weeks, otherwise it's unmanageable.
  C. Is long to allow me to manage a variety of hairstyles depending on my needs so I just make sure the ends are trimmed frequently.

  It gets trimmed depending upon my upcoming parts but I like it to grow as much as possible.

6. My hair color:
  A. Is something I've experimented with myself.
  B. Yuck! Ruin my hair with chemicals?
  C. Is done at the beauty shop every six weeks.

  Is done at the shop when it needs it — this is a little routine in the life of an actress!

7. The colors I wear most frequently are:
  A. Neutrals that mix well in the business world: navy, burgundy, cream, and things that are "safe."
  B. Bright colors, I love 'em.
  C. Whatever the fashion mavens say is "in," as long as it's also flattering to my skin tones.

  Pastels but colorful!

8. For a purse, I usually carry:
  A. One good all-purpose bag that goes with all my clothes.
  B. Something fun and inexpensive that holds all the junk I carry around.
  C. Whatever matches my clothes.

  I often carry two bags — and so much junk!

9. The hair appliances I rely on include:
  A. A round brush and blow-dryer.
  B. I have all kinds of stuff, but I never use it.
  C. Electric rollers, hairpins, combs, clips, curling iron, crimper, dryers, and brushes.

  also electric curlers

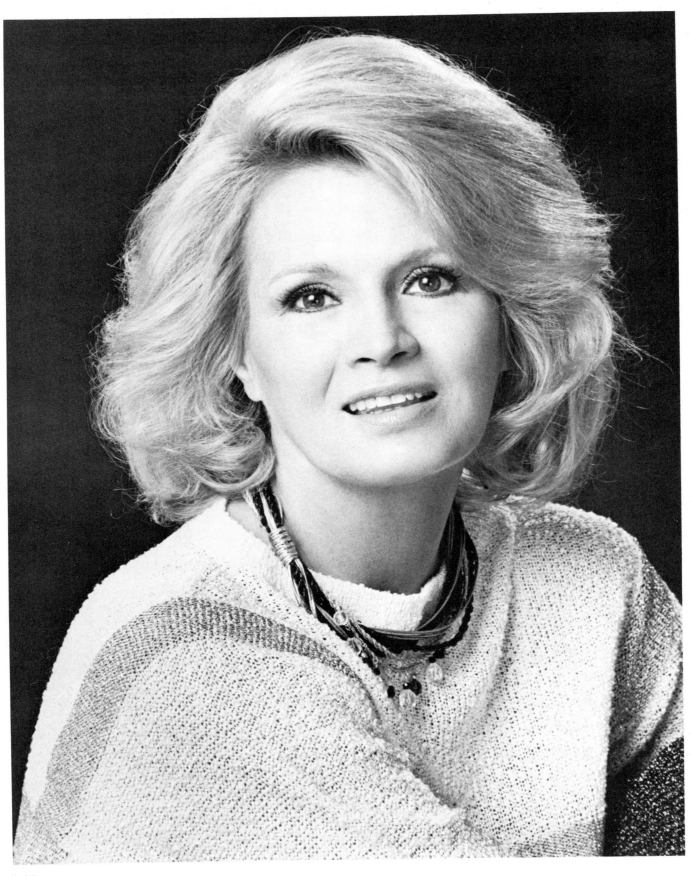

10. **For breakfast, I:**
    A. Grab something on the way to work or eat at my desk
    B. Have cold cereal and fruit.
    C. Eat a light meal if I'm dieting or a little more if I'm having a late lunch.
    D. I have nothing!

11. **When I bathe, I:**
    (A.) Take a shower first thing in the morning.
    B. Take a shower several times a day, after tennis or swimming.
    C. Take a leisurely bath.

12. **I have help in my home:**
    A. Never.
    B. Once or twice a week.
    (C.) Full time.

13. **I put myself together:**
    (A.) To please myself.
    B. To suit my life-style.
    C. To please my man.
    All three.

14. **I work:**
    A. Nine to five at a regular job.
    B. You think taking care of the kids isn't full-time work?
    C. Flexible hours or not at all.

15. **My fingernails:**
    A. Are manicured by me.

B. Are kept short and neat for simplicity.
    C. I have done weekly.
    A and B.

16. **When it comes to athletics:**
    A. Weekends are the only time I have for recreational sports.
    B. I'd only be more active if I were training for the Olympics.
    C. I don't sweat.
    I do them whenever it fits my work schedule!

17. **If I have a little extra money to splurge with, I:**
    A. Buy something I need.
    B. Get something for the kids.
    (C.) Buy something wonderful I've been dying to have.

18. **My idea of the perfect vacation would be to:**
    A. Travel to the major cities of Europe.
    B. Go hiking and backpacking.
    C. Escape to a spa.
    Both A and B.

19. **My bedtime is:**
    A. After the 11:00 P.M. news.
    B. Early, after an exhausting day.
    C. Whenever the party's over.
    early if nothing exciting is on TV.

20. **If I could sum up my beauty routine simply, I would say it's:**
    A. Sensible.
    (B.) Practical.
    C. Time-consuming.
    Practical for everyday wear!

Jose says:
Angie's hair is very fine, so it is cut in one length, to show off her bone structure. The style is sophisticated and sexy at the same time, which I think is in keeping with her image. Yet it's still easy for her to do herself, which is important to her.

Linda Gray

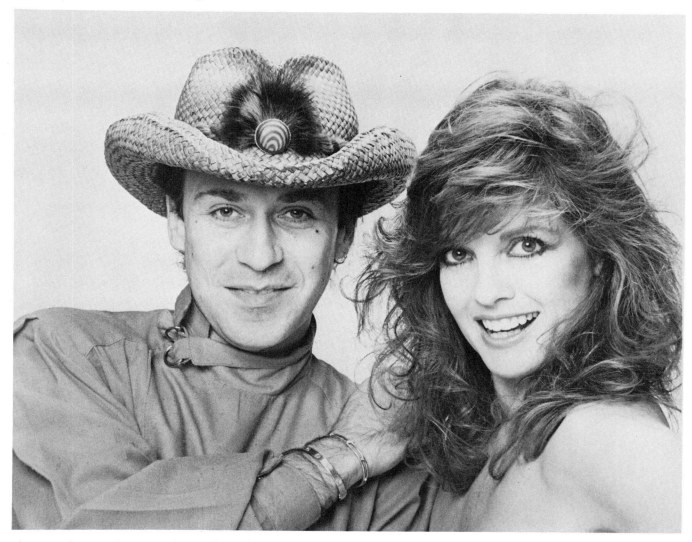

I'm Jose's number-one fan. I heard about him from two of my girl friends. He cuts Victoria Principal's hair and I never thought having him cut hair for two people on the same show about it being a conflict. As soon as Jose saw me, he said, "My God, you're so much younger in person."

Well, you can imagine how I felt! He suggested a body wave, lightening my hair three shades, and a cut, and all I could think was, "I hope he knows what he's doing." Over a period of two weeks we did everything he'd suggested. I hardly had time to think about it—it happened one, two, three. I went from dull to dynamite.

My dark hair made me look older on camera, like a matron. When Jose suggested bangs, I looked at him a bit strangely, but I walked out of his place looking ten years younger—that's a fact. And because of that, my attitude is more up.

Jose has a real sense about women. He loves them, and he knows exactly what's right and what's attractive. I hate cookie-cutter shops. Jose's not like that. Despite all the celebs he does and the fact that he works on two of us from the same show, none of his clients look alike.

As an actress I need enough length to my hair to be able to create different styles. My secret fantasy is to have very short hair, but my character can't take it, so I've given up that dream. Now I want versatility and glamour without looking "done." I like a style that softens my jaw and shows off my eyes and is easy for me to handle myself. And Jose has found all that for me.

JOSE EBER'S LIFE-STYLE QUIZ

Linda Gray

My personality is Red, and that's a fact. I just came out with this score because of my working life.

1. When I wake up in the morning:
A. I look at the alarm clock and panic. I'm already late.
B. Who needs an alarm clock? I'm up with the birds, or the kids, and ready to go.
C. I roll over and go back to sleep for another half hour because last night really was a bit too much.

2. My regular morning routine:
A. Takes no more than half an hour because I'm so busy.
B. Is postponed until later in the day, because I'm out the door for tennis or carpool.
C. Depends on what I'm doing during the day and what's cooking for the upcoming evening.

3. When I look in the mirror each morning I:
A. Wish I had time to do something about what I see.
B. Splash cold water on my face and check the condition of my skin.
C. Study each line, blemish, and soft spot mercilessly, until I'm satisfied I know exactly how to best care for what I've seen.

4. First thing in the morning, my hair:
A. Needs a wash and blow-dry.
B. Kind of falls into place, because my haircut is easy to care for.
C. Is almost perfect, because I just had it done yesterday.

5. My hair:
A. Gets cut whenever I'm in the mood or can't do a thing with it.
B. Needs to be cut every four–six weeks; otherwise it's unmanageable.
C. Is long to allow me to manage a variety of hairstyles depending on my needs so I just make sure the ends are trimmed frequently.

Well, it's B too.

6. My hair color:
A. Is something I've experimented with myself.
B. Yuck! Ruin my hair with chemicals?
C. Is done at the beauty shop every six weeks.

7. The colors I wear most frequently are:
A. Neutrals that mix well in the business world: navy, burgundy, cream, and things that are "safe."
B. Bright colors, I love 'em.
C. Whatever the fashion mavens say is "in," as long as it's also flattering to my skin tones.

I don't like it and I don't "safe" and like "in" things.

8. For a purse, I usually carry:
A. One good all-purpose bag that goes with all my clothes.
B. Something fun and inexpensive that holds all the junk I carry around.
C. Whatever matches my clothes.

9. The hair appliances I rely on include:
A. A round brush and blow-dryer.
B. I have all kinds of stuff, but I never use it.
C. Electric rollers, hairpins, combs, clips, curling iron, crimper, dryers, and brushes.

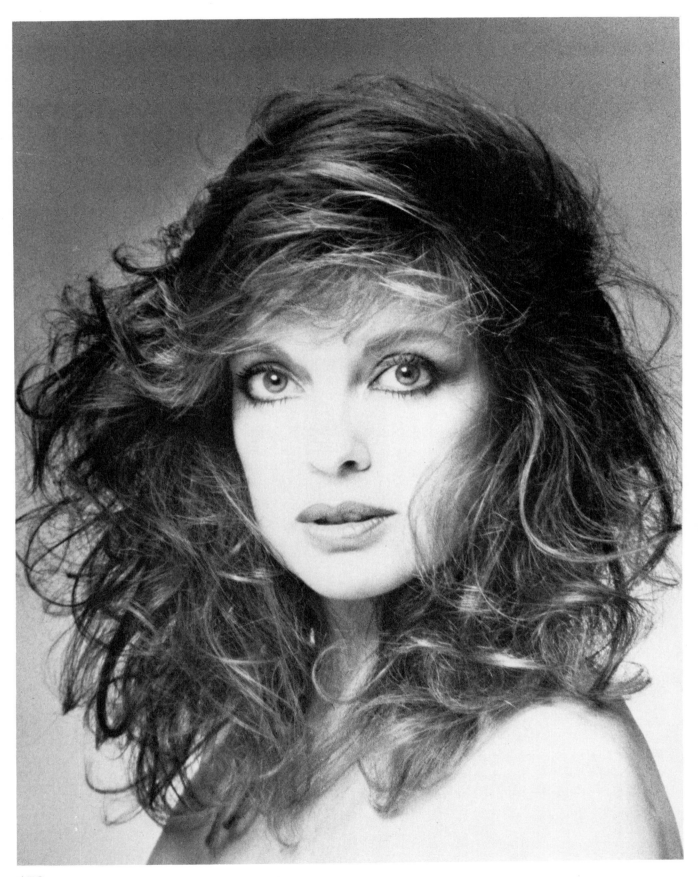

10. For breakfast, I:
  A. Grab something on the way to work or eat at my desk
  B. Have cold cereal and fruit.
  (C.) Eat a light meal if I'm dieting or a little more if I'm having a late lunch.

11. When I bathe, I:
  (A.) Take a shower first thing in the morning.
  B. Take a shower several times a day, after tennis or swimming.
  C. Take a leisurely bath.

12. I have help in my home:
  A. Never.
  B. Once or twice a week.
  (C.) Full time.

13. I put myself together:
  (A.) To please myself.
  B. To suit my life-style.
  C. To please my man.

14. I work:
  A. Nine to five at a regular job.
  B. You think taking care of the kids isn't full-time work?
  C. Flexible hours or not at all.

15. My fingernails:
  A. Are manicured by me.
  B. Are kept short and neat for simplicity.
  (C.) I have done weekly.

16. When it comes to athletics:
  A. Weekends are the only time I have for recreational sports.
  (B.) I'd only be more active if I were training for the Olympics.
  C. I don't sweat.

17. If I have a little extra money to splurge with, I:
  A. Buy something I need.
  B. Get something for the kids.
  (C.) Buy something wonderful I've been dying to have.

18. My idea of the perfect vacation would be to:
  A. Travel to the major cities of Europe.
  B. Go hiking and backpacking.
  (C.) Escape to a spa.

It would be A, but because of the show, it's got to be C. With a weekly show, it's got to be C. I need to rest, not run around looking at museums and cathedrals.

19. My bedtime is:
  A. After the 11:00 P.M. news.
  (B.) Early, after an exhausting day.
  C. Whenever the party's over.

20. If I could sum up my beauty routine simply, I would say it's:
  (A.) Sensible.
  B. Practical.
  C. Time-consuming.

In my heart I'm a Red, I know it!

Jose says:
Right away I gave Linda a side bang, to soften her forehead, which is very attractive but makes her look older. So I like the long bangs for her. This accentuates her incredible eyes. She has such big ones, and now the bangs frame them. I wanted to make her look a little more funky—youthful kind of funky, not as severe as she looked before. After I made the bangs, I layered the top for a little fullness and to give her some body to balance them. Then I sent her upstairs to lighten her color a little bit.

Victoria MacMahon

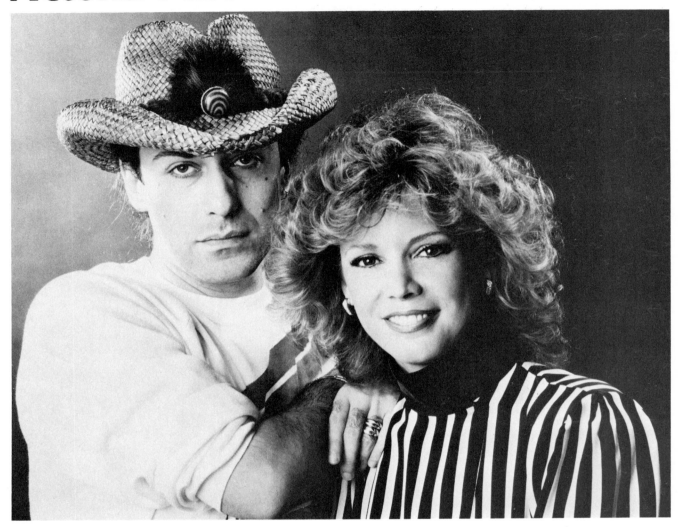

Victoria MacMahon is the wife of Ed MacMahon, and she has a very busy life as a professional wife. Wherever Ed goes, Victoria does too, and she always looks radiant.

Because Victoria will never step out of the house until her hair and makeup are perfect, she takes a lot of time to get the details right. Her hair is very fine, and all her life—since childhood—she's had a permanent. She uses electric rollers every day, so she is very, very careful about her hair condition and makes sure that she does not damage her already fragile hair. Victoria lets her hair dry naturally, so she can avoid using a blow-dryer, which would put more heat on her hair and therefore do more damage. This is a good trick to remember for people who have to use rollers every day.

Victoria has the same needs as a Life-style Green, because once she is dressed, coiffed, and made up for the day, her look has to last and last. She may also be going out in the evening and may not have time to redo her hair and makeup, so she takes extra time in the morning to make sure she looks great, and then doesn't have to worry. Sometimes for the evening she pins her hair up. She does have the kind of hair that could dry naturally and appear finished, but this look would be very casual, and not as sophisticated as she likes. Really, though, she is a Life-style Blue, and feels best with her routine and the knowledge that every hair is in place and will stay there.

JOSE EBER'S LIFE-STYLE QUIZ

Victoria MacMahon

1. **When I wake up in the morning:**
   - A. I look at the alarm clock and panic. I'm already late. *(circled)*
   - B. Who needs an alarm clock? I'm up with the birds, or the kids, and ready to go.
   - C. I roll over and go back to sleep for another half hour because last night really was a bit too much.

2. **My regular morning routine:**
   - A. Takes no more than half an hour because I'm so busy.
   - B. Is postponed until later in the day, because I'm out the door for tennis or carpool.
   - C. Depends on what I'm doing during the day and what's cooking for the upcoming evening. *(circled)*

3. **When I look in the mirror each morning I:**
   - A. Wish I had time to do something about what I see.
   - B. Splash cold water on my face and check the condition of my skin.
   - C. Study each line, blemish, and soft spot mercilessly, until I'm satisfied I know exactly how to best care for what I've seen.
   - D. I don't look at myself in the mirror. I brush my teeth and get into the shower *(handwritten)*

4. **First thing in the morning, my hair:**
   - A. Needs a wash and blow-dry. *(circled)*
   - B. Kind of falls into place, because my haircut is easy to care for.
   - C. Is almost perfect, because I just had it done yesterday.

5. **My hair:**
   - A. Gets cut whenever I'm in the mood or can't do a thing with it.
   - B. Needs to be cut every four–six weeks; otherwise it's unmanageable. *(circled)*
   - C. Is long to allow me to manage a variety of hairstyles depending on my needs so I just make sure the ends are trimmed frequently.

6. **My hair color:**
   - A. Is something I've experimented with myself.
   - B. Yuck! Ruin my hair with chemicals?
   - C. Is done at the beauty shop every six weeks. *(circled)*

7. **The colors I wear most frequently are:**
   - A. Neutrals that mix well in the business world: navy, burgundy, cream, and things that are "safe."
   - B. Bright colors, I love 'em. *(circled)*
   - C. Whatever the fashion mavens say is "in," as long as it's also flattering to my skin tones.

8. **For a purse, I usually carry:**
   - A. One good all-purpose bag that goes with all my clothes.
   - B. Something fun and inexpensive that holds all the junk I carry around.
   - C. Whatever matches my clothes. *(circled)*

9. **The hair appliances I rely on most are:**
   - A. A round brush and blow-dryer.
   - B. I have pounds of stuff I never use
   - C. Electric rollers, hair iron, combs, clips, curling crimper, dryers, and brushes. *(circled)*

(handwritten notes across bottom:) May I make a comment here? My whole life revolves around those hot rollers! When were on the road I'm always waiting for those hot rods! — Ed

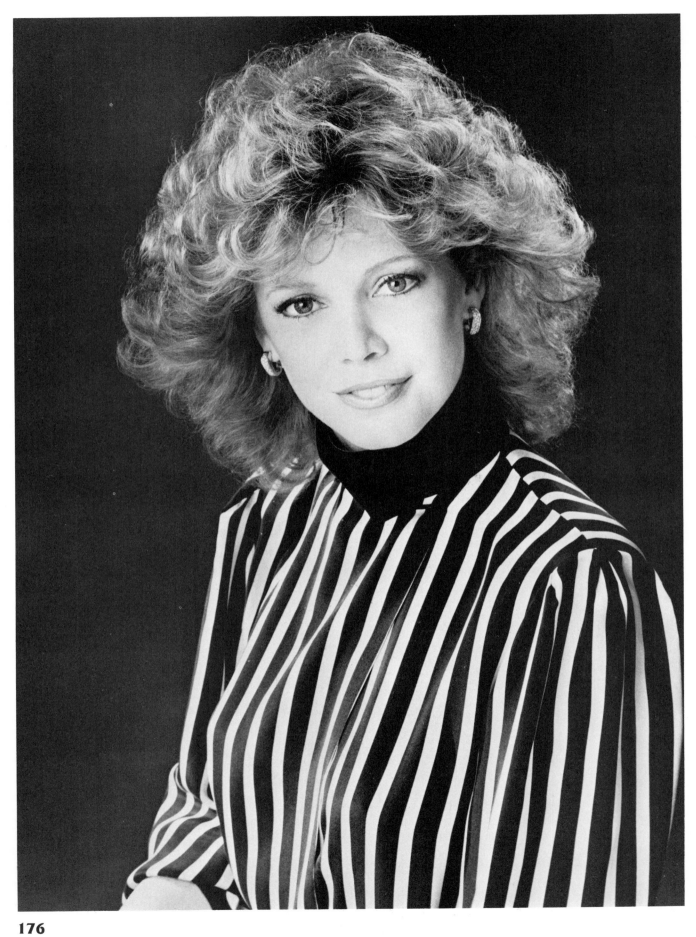

10. **For breakfast, I:**
    A. Grab something on the way to work or eat at my desk
    B. Have cold cereal and fruit.
    C. Eat a light meal if I'm dieting or a little more if I'm having a late lunch.

    None of these. I have coffee and half a grapefruit, every morning

11. **When I bathe, I:**
    (A.) Take a shower first thing in the morning.
    B. Take a shower several times a day, after tennis or swimming.
    C. Take a leisurely bath.

    I shower every morning, but when I have time for a leisurely bath in the evening, I take one.

12. **I have help in my home:**
    A. Never.
    B. Once or twice a week.
    (C.) Full time.

13. **I put myself together:**
    A. To please myself.
    B. To suit my life-style.
    (C.) To please my man.

14. **I work:**
    A. Nine to five at a regular job.
    B. You think taking care of the kids isn't full-time work?
    (C.) Flexible hours or not at all.

15. **My fingernails:**
    A. Are manicured by me.
    B. Are kept short and neat for simplicity.
    (C.) I have done weekly.

16. **When it comes to athletics:**
    A. Weekends are the only time I have for recreational sports.
    (B.) I'd only be more active if I were training for the Olympics.
    C. I don't sweat.

    I do my excercises every night after Ed goes to bed.

17. **If I have a little extra money to splurge with, I:**
    A. Buy something I need.
    (B.) Get something for the kids.
    C. Buy something wonderful I've been dying to have.

    I'd buy something for Ed.

18. **My idea of the perfect vacation would be to:**
    (A.) Travel to the major cities of Europe.
    B. Go hiking and backpacking.
    C. Escape to a spa.

19. **My bedtime is:**
    (A.) After the 11:00 P.M. news.
    B. Early, after an exhausting day.
    C. Whenever the party's over.

20. **If I could sum up my beauty routine simply, I would say it's:**
    A. Sensible.
    B. Practical.
    (C.) Time-consuming.

Jose says:
For Victoria, the hair is swept off the forehead, because it is small, and brushed away at the temples to accentuate her beautiful eyes and cheekbones. Her hair has some length, but the sides and top are shorter, to give her fullness and the swept-away look. She is not the type to wear her hair in a natural style, so she has a permanent and uses electric rollers.

Marilyn McCoo

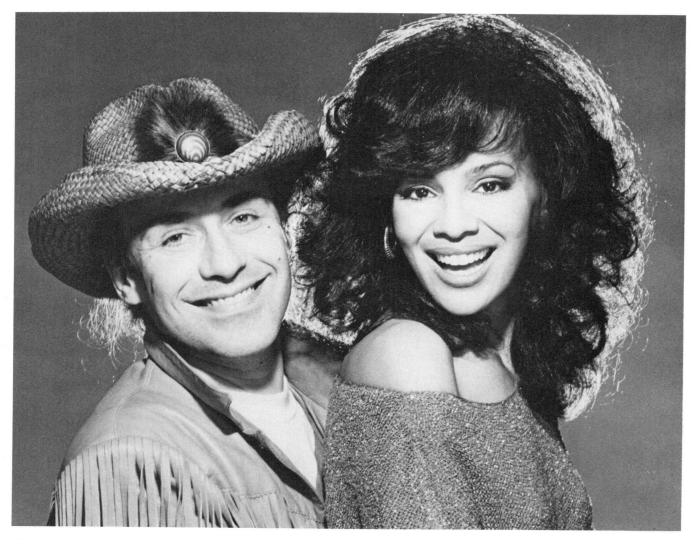

I highly respect my sister's opinion when it comes to beauty, so when she recommended Jose, I went to see him. She pays even more attention to what's going on in this field than I do, so I trust her. My sister had met Jose when she was hosting a noontime talk show in Los Angeles and did a story on him. She started going to him, and then she sent me. She said Jose was the best stylist she had found in this country.

The first time I went to him, he gave me a cut I thought was nice but not special. But afterward, everyone told me how great I looked. Every time Jose cut my hair, it was different, and every time, I got a lot of compliments. So I'm at the point where I really trust him and I don't feel he can do anything wrong.

I've even sent my younger sister to him, so now he's done the whole family. And she claims she's had great results from her cut too. She lives in Washington, D.C., but when she comes to visit she goes to Jose.

I like to keep my hair long, but the ends are damaged and need to be trimmed regularly. I hurt my hair by relaxing it, even though it was done professionally, in a salon, so I'm letting it grow out and having the damage cut out slowly. Jose tells me what I have to do to accomplish this task. We layer it for fullness, and that leaves some length and still lets us cut the damaged part, on the ends.

My face is very thin, so I like to wear my hair in a way that deemphasizes that, and the layers help. I usually like to play down the size of my forehead, too. I don't worry about anything else on my face, because I can't do anything about it.

JOSE EBER'S LIFE-STYLE QUIZ

Marilyn McCoo

1. When I wake up in the morning:

A. I look at the alarm clock and panic. I'm already late. *(circled)*

B. Who needs an alarm clock? I'm up with the birds, or the kids, and ready to go.

C. I roll over and go back to sleep for another half hour because last night really was a bit too much.

2. My regular morning routine:

A. Takes no more than half an hour because I'm so busy.

B. Is postponed until later in the day, because I'm out the door for tennis or carpool.

C. Depends on what I'm doing during the day and what's cooking for the upcoming evening. *(circled)*

Handwritten: I'm so slow, no matter what my morning routine is so busy I'm still running late.

3. When I look in the mirror each morning I:

A. Wish I had time to do something about what I see. *(circled)*

B. Splash cold water on my face and check the condition of my skin.

C. Study each line, blemish, and soft spot meticulously, until I'm satisfied I know exactly how to best care for what I've

Handwritten: I don't have time for this, because I'm so slow.

4. First thing in the morning, my hair:

A. Needs a wash and blow-dry.

B. Kind of falls into place, because my haircut is easy to care for. *(circled)*

C. Is almost perfect, because I just had it done yesterday.

5. My hair:

A. Get cut whenever I'm in the mood or can't do a thing with it.

B. Needs to be cut every four to six weeks; otherwise it's unmanageable.

C. Is long to allow me to manage a variety of hairstyles depending on my needs so I just make sure the ends are trimmed frequently. *(circled)*

Handwritten: It's sort of C, but Jose trims it every six to eight weeks and does something a little different with it.

6. My hair color:

A. Is something I've experimented with myself.

B. Yuck. Ruin my hair with chemicals?

C. Is done at the beauty shop every six weeks. *(circled)*

Handwritten: It's my own hair color right now. I had ruined my hair before, so I'm really careful now. And if I ever have my hair chemically treated. But whatever I have done to my hair, it's always by a professional.

7. The colors I wear most frequently:

A. Neutrals that mix well in the business world: navy, burgundy, cream, and things that are "safe." *(circled)*

B. Bright colors. I love 'em.

C. Whatever the fashion mavens say is "in" and as long as it's also flattering.

Handwritten: I wear colors that look good against my skin. I love neutrals, but I have color moods. I was on a purple kick for a few years, now I'm moving into red and gray, mostly for accent.

8. For a purse, I usually carry:

A. One good all-purpose bag that goes with all my clothes. *(circled)*

B. Something fun and inexpensive that holds all the junk I carry around.

C. Whatever matches my clothes.

9. The hair appliances I rely on include:

A. A round brush and blow-dryer.

B. I have all kinds of stuff, but I never use it. *(circled)*

C. Electric rollers, hairpins, combs, clips, curling iron, crimper, dryers, and brushes.

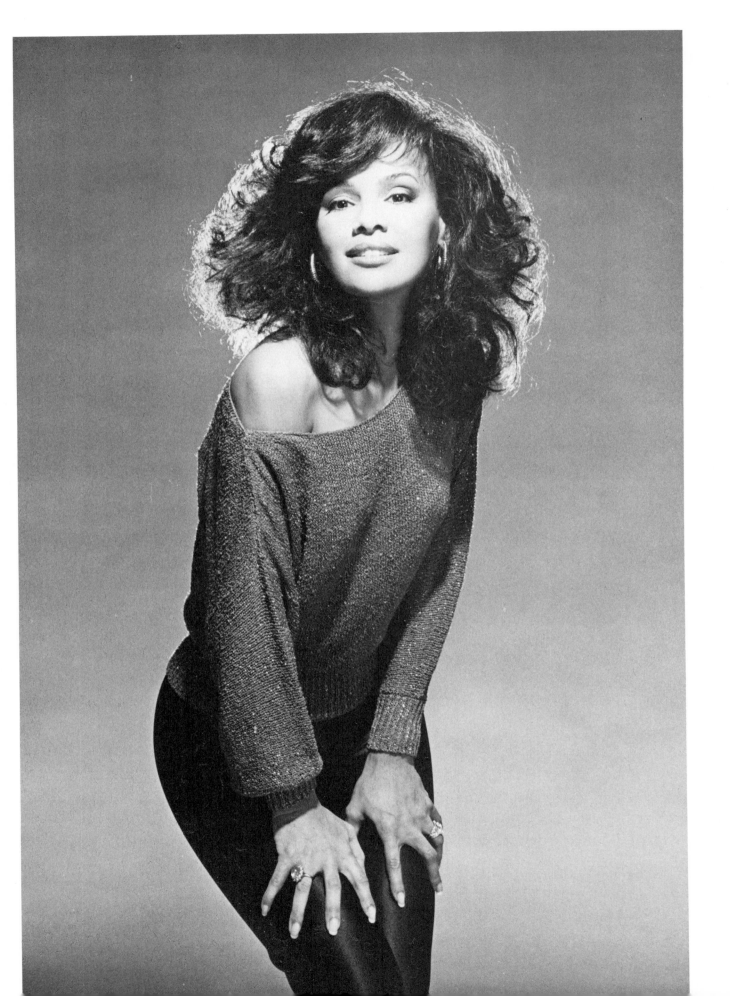

10. **For breakfast, I:**
    A. Grab something on the way to work or eat at my desk
    B. ⓑ Have cold cereal and fruit
    C. Eat a light meal of eggs, dieting or a little more if I'm having a late lunch.

    I eat a big hot breakfast... and sausage or cold cereal. I have no lunch. If I'm having lunch, I'll skip breakfast

11. **When I bathe, I:**
    A. Ⓐ Take a shower first thing in the morning.
    B. Take a shower several times a day, after tennis or swimming.
    C. Take a leisurely bath.

12. **I have help in my home:**
    A. Never.
    B. Once or twice a week.
    C. Ⓒ Full time.

13. **I put myself together:**
    A. Ⓐ To please myself.
    B. To suit my life-style.
    C. To please my man.

    It's all of them really.

14. **I work:**
    A. Nine to five at a regular job.
    B. You think taking care of the kids isn't full-time work?
    C. Flexible hours or not at all.

15. **My fingernails:**
    A. Are manicured by me.
    B. Are kept short and neat for simplicity.
    C. Ⓒ I have done weekly.

    And I keep them short.

16. **When it comes to athletics:**
    A. Ⓐ Weekends are the only time I have for recreational sports
    B. I'd only like to be more active if I were training for the Olympics.
    C. I don't see...

    I would like to have more time but when I'm working, I don't. Sometimes I can sneak in a game of tennis during the week, but not often.

17. **If I have a little extra money to splurge with, I:**
    A. Buy something I need.
    B. Get something for the kids.
    C. Ⓒ Buy something wonderful I've been dying to have.

18. **My idea of the perfect vacation would be to:**
    A. Ⓐ Travel to the major cities of Europe.
    B. Go hiking and backpacking.
    C. Escape to a spa.

19. **My bedtime is:**
    A. Ⓐ After the 11:00 P.M. news.
    B. Early after an exhausting day.
    C. Whenever the movie's over.

    More or less. I usually fall asleep watching television during news or late movies or anything after the news.

20. **If I could sum up my beauty routine simply, I would say it's:**
    A. Sensible.
    B. Practical.
    C. Ⓒ Time-consuming.

    It's sensible in terms of my needs, but there's no doubt that it's time-consuming. I have sensitive skin, and if I don't take time with it, I won't be able to wear makeup, so I'm very careful. I guess that means all three answers are true.

Jose says:
Marilyn needs a little height to balance her hairstyle, so the top is layered. She keeps it long so she can have different styles, and has a lot of fullness because her hair is naturally curly. She has it relaxed in the salon so it doesn't control her, but it still has good body and fullness.

Pia Zadora

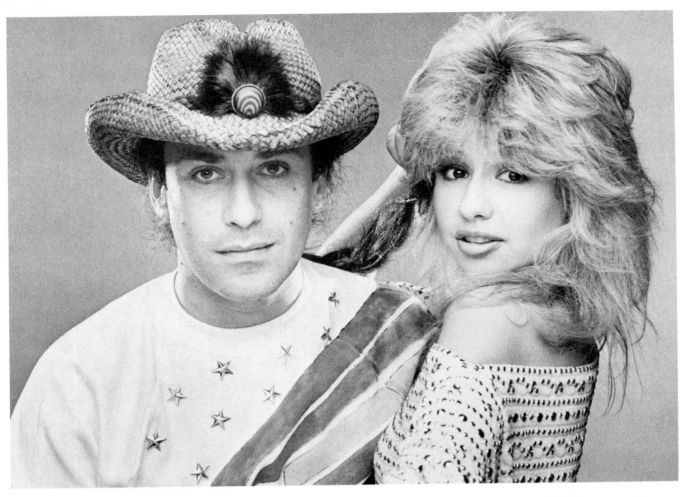

I adore Jose. I think he's the greatest. He's the classiest guy in the business, and he's got real soul. I trust him so much that he's become part of my family. My mother calls him "Exotic Jose" because of the way he looks, but she always catches him on television.

My biggest problem with my appearance is that everyone thinks I look so young. Actually, I seem younger now than I did five years ago. I got married young, and I was trying so hard to look older. But as you age, you develop your own taste and your own looks, you learn you don't have to fit any mold, and that what others think is just not that important. Once I had a sense of myself, my real look started to develop. I met Jose right after that.

I was about to start a picture called *Butterfly*, and I think it was the director who said I needed to appear different and sent me to Jose. Now I've found the way I want to be. I also have an attitude about how I want to look. And Jose helps me. I like to be able to go to extremes. One night I might like to wear long eyelashes and fancy jewelry and curls, and the next night I might wear a t-shirt, a mini, and really shaggy hair. That's what keeps me from being boring.

Obviously I need hair that I can fix however I want. And that's Jose's department.

JOSE EBER'S LIFE-STYLE QUIZ

Pia Zadora

1. **When I wake up in the morning:**
   A. I look at the alarm clock and panic, then I'm already late.
   B. Who needs an alarm clock? I'm up except the birds, or the kids are ready to go.
   C. I roll over and go back to sleep for another half hour because last night really was a bit too much.

   alarm clocks are out. Someone. It's hard to get me up. makes my place. When I'm working, then the Studio calls me. When I finally get up, the first things I say is "Where is the telephone!"

2. **My regular morning routine:**
   A. Takes no more than half an hour because I'm so busy.
   B. Is postponed until later and the carpool.
   C. Depends on what I'm doing during the day and what's cooking for the upcoming evening.

   In California, it's up and exercise for an hour, jump in the jacuzzi for fifteen minutes, then into the steam shower and then throw on my jeans. In New York it's the same, without the jacuzzi.

3. **When I look in the mirror each morning I:**
   A. Wish I had time to do something about what I see.
   B. Splash cold water on my face and check the condition of my skin.
   C. Study each line, blemish, and soft spot mercilessly, until I'm satisfied I know exactly how to best cover what I've seen.

   It's not really C. But I look every day waiting for the lines to come.

4. **First thing in the morning, my hair:**
   A. Needs a wash and blow-dry.
   B. Kind of falls into place, because my haircut is easy to care for.
   C. Is almost perfect, because I just had it done yesterday.

5. **My hair:**
   A. Gets cut whenever I'm in the mood or can't do a thing with it.
   B. Needs to be cut every four–six weeks; otherwise it's unmanageable.
   C. Is long to allow me to manage a variety of hairstyles depending on need, and I just make sure the ends are trimmed frequently.

   It's cut every three weeks and grows like a tropical jungle. My nails too.

6. **My hair color:**
   A. Is something I've experimented with myself.
   B. Yuck! Ruin my hair with chemicals?
   C. Is done at the beauty shop every six weeks.

   I don't talk about my hair color or my age.

7. **The colors I wear most frequently are:**
   A. Neutrals that mix well in the business world: navy, burgundy, cream, and things that are "safe."
   B. Bright colors, I love them!
   C. Whatever the fashion mavens say.

   whatever I'm in the mood for. It could be dazzle and glitter or taupes. I like to express a change of mood with a change of clothing.

8. **For a purse, I usually carry:**
   A. One good all-purpose bag that goes with all my clothes.
   B. Something fun and inexpensive that holds all the junk I carry around.
   C. Whatever matches my clothes.

   For the evening it's C.

9. **The hair appliances I rely on include:**
   A. A round brush and blow-dryer.
   B. I have all kinds of stuff, but I never use it.
   C. Electric rollers, hairpins, combs, clips, curling iron, crimper, dryers, and brushes.

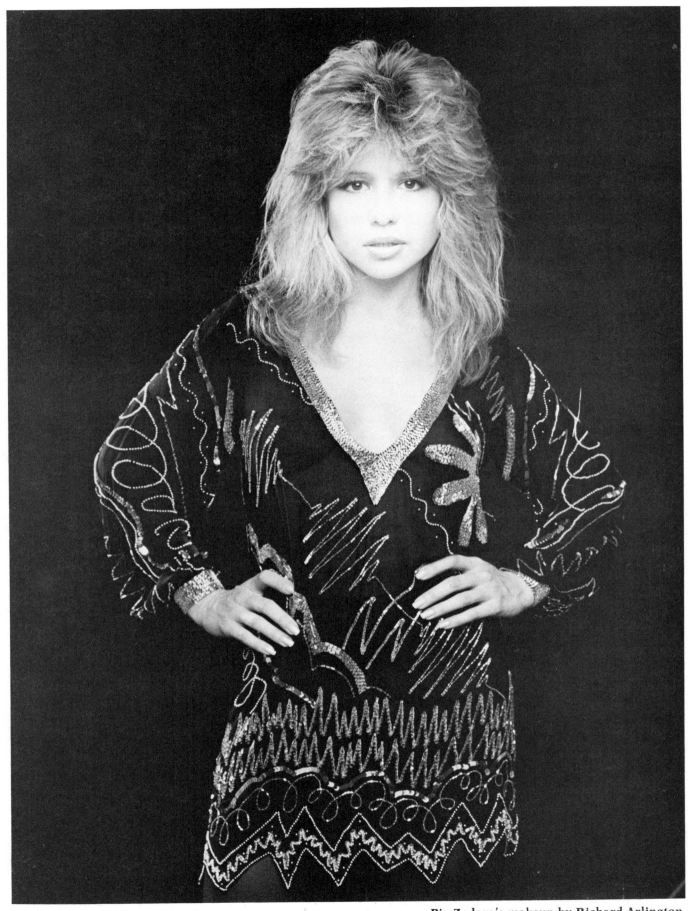

Pia Zadora's makeup by Richard Arlington.

10. **For breakfast, I:**
    A. Grab something on the way to work or eat at my desk
    B. Have cold cereal and fruit.
    C. Eat a light meal if I'm dieting or a little more if I'm having a late lunch.
    Herb tea and a piece of fruit.

11. **When I bathe, I:**
    A. Take a shower first thing in the morning.
    B. Take a shower several times a day, after tennis or swimming.
    C. Take a leisurely bath.
    In relaxing.

12. **I have help in my home:**
    A. Never.
    B. Once or twice a week.
    C. Full time.
    They call me the tornado. I need someone to go from room to room after me.

13. **I put myself together:**
    A. To please myself.
    B. To suit my life-style.
    C. To please my man.
    You can't please anyone unless you please yourself.

14. **I work:**
    A. Nine to five at a regular job.
    B. You think taking care of the kids isn't full-time work?
    C. Flexible hours or not at all.

15. **My fingernails:**
    A. Are manicured by me.
    They're done weekly if I have a chance, but I'll do them myself if I have to. Sometimes I do them at dinner or on an airplane.

    B. Are kept short and neat for simplicity.
    C. have done weekly.

16. **When it comes to athletics:**
    A. Weekends are the only time I have for recreational sports.
    B. I'd only be more active if I were training for the Olympics.
    C. I don't [go?] into competitive
    I'm not into competitive sports, but I ride horseback, I run on the beach, and do exercises at home.

17. **If I have a little extra money to splurge with, I:**
    A. Buy something I need.
    B. Get something for the kids.
    C. Buy something wonderful I've been dying to have.

18. **My idea of the perfect vacation would be to:**
    A. Travel to the major cities of Europe.
    B. Go hiking and backpacking.
    C. Escape to a spa.
    I have a spa in my own home, that's the best escape.

19. **My bedtime is:**
    A. After the 11:00 P.M. news.
    B. Early, after an exhausting day.
    C. Whenever the party's over.

20. **If I could sum up my beauty routine simply, I would say it's:**
    A. Sensible.
    B. Practical.
    C. Time-consuming.

Jose says:
Pia has a very small face and is extremely petite, so we make her a little bigger with big, messy hair. She can wear it many ways, but when it dries naturally, it has a wild, sexy look.

Part Four:

THE RESULTS

So, darling, here we are. We have all the pieces; we've seen how some of my clients coordinate their life-styles with their hairstyles. Now it's your turn.

We are going to find the right look for you, and you alone. Since I am here and you are there, how can we do this? It's simple. Together we are going to talk to your hairstylist.

The purpose of this book is to help you to find a style that you love, that suits your life, and that also fits the variables in it. You are not supposed to be cutting out pictures of the stars and running to the bathroom with your hot rollers, trying to make yourself look like them. Nor are you supposed to take their pictures to your hairstylist and say, "See, here, my friend, I'm a Life-style Red, and so is Ali MacGraw. Make me look like her."

This is what you should do.

• Be sure of your life-style category. You may want to retest. If you have some questions or if you think you fall into two of the categories, remember:

•   Reds are sporty and have no time for anything.

•   Greens have a set amount of time once a day for hair and beauty.

•   Blues have as much time as they need.

•   If you tested in one category but this oversimplification puts you in another, you may want to study both categories and make a change. Then pick the Life-style classification that best suits you.

• Go over your section of the book again, this time just looking at the pictures and picking up on the Life-style clues in the interviews and quizzes. Separate the stars from their glamour and learn how they coordinate their looks. Check the variables in the face picture against your own face. On the chart on the next page, fill in the parts of your face that are most like the ones you see in the pictures.

• Be sure you have filled in all the worksheets in this book: you should have a Life-style Quiz, a Personal Worksheet, and the Check-off Chart filled in with as much detail and honesty as possible. More information is better than less.

• Once everything is filled out, call your hairstylist—or even call a new unknown one. Speak to him personally, not to the receptionist, and explain that you need a hairstyle to fit your life-style. Tell him you have filled out the worksheets in my book and would like to show him your answers and scores and work with him to find a new style for you. If the hairstylist says that this is the craziest thing he has ever heard of, hang up, darling. If he won't listen to your ideas or discuss your opinions and look at information that will help him to make you prettier and happier, then you can imagine what he will do to your hair—whatever he wants! One of the reasons I am so successful, I swear to you, is that I *listen* to what *all* my clients say to me— every single one. I may expand on their ideas, but I never go beyond what they say they want.

• Study all the pictures and interviews carefully. Not all the women here are celebrities. Some of them have a life-style just like yours, whether you are Red, Green, or Blue. Look carefully at their faces, and consider their Life-style quizzes and profiles and the hairstyles I've selected for them. Then chart again the similarities to your own face and life-style.

What you are doing is gathering ammunition. It's like doing your homework. You are going off to do battle for your face and your future good looks. You need to be well prepared, with the kind of information that will get you maximum results.

I get letters from women all over the country—phone calls, too. Most of the writers say they are saving all their money to come to Beverly Hills to see me. (One woman called me to say she just knew that if I cut her hair, her husband wouldn't leave her!) I think this is very flattering, but it is not necessary. You can get the kind of haircut you need in your hometown. Your hairstylist just might need a little help. You probably will get a classic haircut, and this simply needs to be executed properly. You need a good haircut, don't get me wrong, but it has to be combined with your other life-style variables, to give you more—a great hairstyle.

So the point is to find the *right* haircut for you, not the stylist who cuts hair better than anyone else in your neighborhood. Most people don't live in Beverly Hills, New York, Paris, or Tokyo. Yet they still have the ability to look as good as the women who live in those cities and go to some of the best hairdressers in the world.

The cut is very important, but pairing the right cut with the right hairstyle is what's going to make you the happiest. You may have to try several stylists and haircuts before you find what works best for you, your hair, and your life-style.

So don't feel stranded, darling. It's not you off there, with me out here in Beverly Hills, unable to help you. The psychiatrist leads you to find the answers to your problems yourself. Well, I have given you the information you need to find a hairstylist who can make you prettier.

We are all in partnership—you, me, and whatever hairstylist you choose as the technician to execute the choices you have made.

CHECK-OFF CHART

You've studied the faces of and beauty facts about women. Some of them are celebrities; others are not. In trying to choose the looks that are right for you and your lifestyle, go back through the book and pick out the aspects of other women's hair and hairstyles that you think will apply to you. Fill in this chart and then show it to your hairstylist.

Life-style _____ (Red, Green, Blue)

My life-style coincides most with:

_____ (fill in the name) _____ (page)

_____   _____

_____   _____

My hair type is the same as or similar to:

_____ (fill in the name) _____ (page)

_____   _____

_____   _____

My face shape and structure are similar to:

_____ (fill in the name) _____ (page)

_____   _____

_____   _____

It's not that I want to look just like her, but I get a good feeling from the way she looks:

_____ (fill in the name) _____ (page)

_____   _____

_____   _____

Life-style Red

HOW TO TALK TO YOUR HAIRSTYLIST

It's very important that you understand that I do not have to cut your hair for you to look great. No matter where you live—in a big city or a small town—you can get a good cut for your face, your life-style, and the variables that matter to you. You just have to know how to do it.

I find Life-Style Reds have a tendency to get short, short haircuts, because they mistakenly think that short hair is easy to care for. Reds aren't usually the kind of people who go berserk if their hair isn't cut exactly the way they want it, because they know they will have it cut again in a matter of weeks. They tend to find a hairstylist they like and stay with him for a while, until they get bored, and then they move on—their loyalty lasts about a year or two. Life-style Greens often change hairdressers every time they need a haircut, and Life-style Blues may stay with the same stylist for fifteen years. Reds are true—for a little while. Short, short hair can be very boring, and that is reason enough to keep changing hairstylists. So here's my suggestion to you, Ms. Life-style Red: talk to your hairstylist about another hair length. I think medium-length hair is much better for the Red woman, possibly with a permanent. The best way to find out is to call your hairstylist. Make an appointment for a consultation. Or try a new hairstylist, but make the appointment to talk first— then decide whether you're ready to cut or go along with his opinion.

If the hairstylist you call does not want to talk first, he's wrong for you. Or if, once you arrive for the consultation, he won't listen to what you say or tells you he only cuts hair the way he wants to—leave immediately. The right hairstylist is one who is willing to work with you so you are both happy. After all, when you leave the salon, it's still your hair. He (or she) won't have to live with it (or you).

Bring this book to the consultation. Show you hairstylist your worksheets and Life-style Quiz. Talk to him about the way you live and the way your hair must perform. Show him your priority list. Make suggestions; ask for his opinion and advice. Talk about alternatives to very short hair—believe me, the Life-style Red woman does not need to have such a short cut if she doesn't want to. When you decide on a cut or a style, make sure you also talk about ways to dress it up at night or for special occasions. Life-style Reds often complain that they hate their hairstyle when it's time to go dancing.

Don't let your stylist try to pressure you into anything. If he does, he's not the right person for you. You may want to think about your consultation and then come back for the cut or restyling later, or you may want to go ahead right on the spot. Some people like to have consultations with different stylists until they find someone they feel is simpatico. This is not a bad idea, because if you find someone you really trust, you might not be tempted to change hairstylists so often.

Discuss conditioning and care with your stylist before you leave. As a Life-style Red you probably aren't using hair spray, hot rollers, or teasing your hair too much. But if you hair is colored, permed, or both, you still need to take care of its condition. A once-a-month condition checkup by your hair expert will take less than a minute and will ensure that your hair always looks its best.

YOUR HAIRCUT

Although the Life-style Red woman is often inclined to get a short haircut, this is not a must, darling. The Life-style Red, like every other woman, can wear any length if it is becoming and flattering. Likewise, you can choose your cut and style. Your hairstylist will be able to help you to choose the *style* that best flatters your face. But think about these alternatives in picking the Life-style Red haircut that's just for you.

Short hair: Short hair is great for an active Red woman *if* your face picture looks good with short hair. But your shoulders shouldn't be too wide or heavy, your neck shouldn't be too long or thick, and you should not look like a man with the style you pick. Hair can always be soft and sexy, even when you are active and in need of wash-and-wear hair. Avoid severe, geometric, and "pixie"-style haircuts if your face isn't perfect (whose is?). Short hair should still be long enough to be versatile—you should be able to use electric rollers or tissue rollers if you want to. Remember, it's the Life-style Red who gets the most bored with her hair when it only has one look, and that kind of short hair is the hardest to dress up. Short hair is usually layered for fullness and the ability to hold style and can be permed, unless it is naturally curly. Naturally curly hair should be cut to follow the curl.

Medium-length hair: I happen to like medium-length hair the most for the Life-style Red woman, because I think it can be worn in the greatest number of ways by the greatest variety of face shapes. Medium-length hair can be layered or cut more or less one length. If you have perfectly straight hair, one length will wash and wear. If your hair has any curl or wave, a layered cut will be easier to control. Wash-and-wear hairstyles must dry naturally and look right for all occasions. If you have no time to blow-dry your hair or use electric rollers, you will not want your hair to dry perfectly. So the cut must be determined by your hair type.

If you do have straight hair, you can change the look with a permanent. The days of stick-straight hair are over, and there is no reason to have boring hair that can only be pulled back.

With medium-length hair you can have layers and the actual hair style cut into your hair as you need them, and can rely on a fashionable look that can be finger-combed for convenience and lasting good looks. No matter how many times you shower or change your clothes or how much you sweat, you can still restore your hairstyle with a minimum of effort.

Long hair: For women with very straight hair who do not live in a cold climate, long hair is a possibility. If their hair can dry naturally and fall in place, then they have enough length for versatility and can always pull back their hair for sports. When long hair has layers cut into it, it dries more quickly and has more body and style. The hair can be permed or cut to natural curl. The only problem with long hair for Life-style Reds is that it takes a long time to dry, and if you live in a cold climate, it can really slow you down.

FINGER-STYLING

The perfect hairstyle for the Life-style Red is one that dries naturally and needs almost no care but still looks great all the time. Does such a hairstyle exist? Absolutely. And the way to guarantee that it dries perfectly and stays that way is to give yourself five to ten minutes in front of the mirror to finger-style. Essentially you will be using your fingers to put your hair in place so that it dries the way it should—and once it's dry, it will stay that way until the next wet-down or sweat-down.

To finger-style:

1. Make sure your haircut is a good one and is not out of shape. An outgrown hairstyle will not finger-style well.
2. Towel-dry your hair for a few minutes to take the extra moisture out. Do this after you shampoo or wet your hair with a spritzer bottle or shower nozzle. Just make sure your hair is no longer sopping wet.
3. If you have a hand dryer, dry and fluff your hair at the roots for about two minutes—this is just to take moisture out and is not a must. It will speed up the drying process if it is convenient for you. Many athletic clubs, spas, or gyms have dryers on the premises for everyone's use. Otherwise, just be sure the towel-drying has absorbed most of the moisture.
4. Run your fingers (use both hands—it's okay) through your hair and casually shape it. This will cause any excess moisture to fall off and will detangle and get the hair in place. You may have to do this several times. If there are serious tangles, get them out with a wide-tooth comb—gently.
5. Once your hair is combed through, you will be able to style it with your fingers and palm. If your hair is one length, work your fingers from underneath your hair and comb out from the hairline to give your hair some lift and body. If your hair is cut in layers, style it by sections. Comb through a section of hair with the fingers of one hand and then squeeze out extra moisture with the palm of that hand. After being squeezed, your hair will be semiwaved. Let it dry naturally. If you can't reach the back to style it, fluff from underneath and squeeze.
6. After your hair is finger-styled, remember that it's still wet, darling. Don't put on your tennis hat or a sweatband. Let your hair dry naturally. Then you can accessorize it however you want to.

NIGHT LIFE

Of the three life-styles, Reds are the least versatile in terms of their hair. Since they are sporty, active people, they only complain about this when a special occasion comes up or they are going out at night and want to look like Rapunzel instead of Tracy Austin.

But don't despair, dear Lady Red. There are a few tricks that will make you happy. First of all, although I know I keep coming back to this, the longer your hair, the more versatile it will be. So if you don't have short, short hair, you might not even face this problem.

If you do have short, short hair and you want to dress it up, here a few things you can do:

• Use a hair accessory—a headband, a flower, a barrette, a comb . . . or even a tiara! What's made you bored and uncomfortable about your night look is that you appear so sensible during the day. Reds are practical, because their life-style demands it. So their evening look will feel that much more special if it is unique. Dare to be a little different, and you will feel better about yourself and your personal style. A band of black velvet ribbon tied in a big bow at the side of your face will be feminine and flattering. Buy two yards of ribbon in the dime store for less than two dollars. (But do iron it each time you use it.) Or buy a silk—or real—flower (coordinate its color with your clothes) and place it at your temple. If your dress has a fabric belt, consider using it as a hair accessory. Remember that earrings are a hair accessory when you have short short hair.

• Use hair gel or styling lotion and finger-style your hair into a more dramatic mode. Slick your hair back, create a few big curls, look like Rod Stewart. Be adventuresome.

• If your hair has any length at all, you can probably make pin curls, which will add some curl and fluff to your regular style. This does take some time and a little planning ahead, but for the right occasion you'll probably enjoy looking different.

Life-style Green

HOW TO TALK TO YOUR HAIRSTYLIST

Women who test Life-style Green seem to get the most frustrated with their hairdressers. They go from one hairstylist to another, never talking about what they really want and hoping that sooner or later they will be happy. Their life-style makes a lot of demands on their hair, and they may not have conveyed their problems clearly to their stylist. Or they may lead such busy lives that a haircut becomes a matter of chance, and they take an appointment wherever they can get it, because instant gratification is more important to them than waiting for a certain stylist.

I think Life-style Greens would be happier if they found a stylist they liked, made a standing appointment every two months or so, and made themselves go. Having a series of consultations with stylists may be a good way to start. Then make a mental agreement to work with the person you choose rather than move on to the next one.

Tell your hairstylist about your Life-style and needs. Show him your quiz, your priority list, and your worksheets. Together you should come up with a style that is flattering and lasts, even considering the variables of your hair and job.

Talk about body and the ways you can get it—with a permanent, setting lotion on the roots, a haircut that's made to hold. You should not be teasing and spraying your hair to make it last all day. The right haircut, the right hairstyle, and the right amount of help (from a permanent, for instance) will give you the results you need.

The Life-style Green woman needs the most individual care, to make sure that her chosen hairstyle will last, so be certain your hairstylist gives you the attention you need and answers whatever questions you may have. Life-style Greens often rush out the door with a quick, "Thank you very much," even when they are dissatisfied with their haircuts. Communication is very important for this life-style. The Green Lady should take the time to talk seriously with her hairstylist. You may have to try a few techniques to find a style that you like and that lasts. But you can do it. You do not need to jump on an airplane and come out to see me.

YOUR HAIRCUT

The most important thing a good Life-style Green haircut can do is to last all day. This is one of its functions. More than any other, the Life-style Green woman needs a good haircut that is right for her. And she must be careful to maintain it so that it does not get out of shape.

Short hair: Short hair that is becoming to the Green woman can be very practical when it is cut in layers, possibly permed, and shaped to flatter and to stay. Short hair dries quickly (which is an asset to the woman who has only a little time for her beauty routine) and is easily styled. It responds well to a curling iron, so you can save time and the health of your hair by using it instead of electric rollers. And short hair that is layered and styled properly will stay longer. Do not pick short hair, darling, if it is not right for your face picture. Short hair is harder to wear than medium-length.

Medium-length hair: Medium-length hair gives the Life-style Green the best chance to flatter her face, and to make optical illusions if necessary. It is also a good length for a woman who is making a dramatic change in her looks—giving up long, hippie-type straight hair, for instance. Medium-length hair is safe, and darling, if security is what you need—then take it.

For your hair to last all day, it should be layered. It doesn't have to be permed, depending on the Green woman's hair type. Hair with a lot of body, when cut properly in layers, should not need it. But a perm offers more than just body, and if you want curls or waves, they add to the ease of your morning routine.

When layered and permed, medium-length hair also grows out easily, without giving you any of the traumas usually associated with it. It doesn't need the same rigorous maintenance a short style does to stay in shape. As long as the layers are properly cut, the shape will remain even as the hair grows. This is good for the working woman who may be juggling so many things that she is a week or two late for her regular haircut. She cannot go for a month—darling, that would be a big mistake—but with medium-length hair, she has a little extra freedom.

Long hair: I think that long hair is more trouble than it is worth for the Life-style Green woman unless she has a perm or her hair is easy to care for. If the hair needs to be curled with rollers every day, this will put pressure on the Life-style Green, because her time is so limited in the morning. So shorter (probably medium-length) hair is better for her. Long hair for the Life-style Green probably should also be layered rather than cut one length, with shorter layers on top and the bulk of the length in back. This allows the hair to have shape and body and to stay all day.

Long straight hair does not have the fashion pizzaz that a working woman needs and is probably not too professional-looking, unless the woman is very young. While long hair can be worn by any age group, long straight hair looks best on women under twenty-five.

NIGHT LIFE

Most Life-style Greens don't even check their hair or change their clothes as they make the passage from day to night. If they are going out or doing something a little special, they often look in the mirror and moan. They don't have time for hot rollers (or the energy, for that matter—they've been working all day!) and they're bored with what they see. Even if their hair is perfect, they are bored.

A small hair accessory like a comb or two is an easy way to perk up hair that may have fallen a bit during the day. An evening hat or a veil is sometimes fun if you are searching for something exotic. Or a little teasing and refluffing may just do the trick.

Usually a good haircut lasts the whole day and looks fine for evening, and the Life-style Green woman is reacting to the fact that she has no time to change her hairstyle rather than that there's something wrong with it. Believe me, darling, anyone whose hairstyle can last all day and through the night should be thrilled and not expect anything more.

I always suggest to the Life-style Green woman that she keep what I call the "P.M. kit" in her handbag or desk drawer. It should include some makeup, a little bottle of fragrance, and maybe some hair combs, or a small, plug-in-anywhere, electric-roller set that can perk up any hairstyle in just a few minutes.

Life-style Blue

HOW TO TALK TO YOUR HAIRSTYLIST

As a Life-style Blue, you should either be thrilled with what you look like at this very moment, or searching for a new hairstylist. Since you have the time and money to do whatever you want, you have no reason not to look your best. If you suffer from Blue Rut, begin to consult with other hairstylists to find someone new. If you're happy with your stylist, bring this to him. Show him your quiz, your worksheets, and your priority lists. Talk them over; then go through the variable lists and make sure you're happy. If there are possibilities you have been ignoring, explore them together. Don't feel that just because you have been wearing your hair a certain way for so many years, it is necessarily the best for you or that you can't change to something else.

Perhaps you can look younger (think of Linda Gray), or more sophisticated, or you'd like to try something completely new. You've got the time, so go ahead. And don't forget about versatility. If your hair has any length, there are probably several styles you can wear successfully. Discover them together with your hairstylist. Get him to teach you how to do some of them yourself. Hair rolling may be too difficult, but you can learn to do tissue-paper rolling and give yourself an added dimension whenever you feel like it.

Be sure to discuss your hair condition at the same time. Blues have a tendency to overwork their hair—what with permanents, coloring, and lots of hot rollers—so make sure you get a hair checkup and a prescription for whatever health aids you need.

You should be able to satisfy all your needs with one haircut, so spend the time going over the worksheets and priority lists and getting your hairstylist to give you his opinion about a variety of styles. You can have everything, so there is no reason to look less than your best.

YOUR HAIRCUT

The only requirement of the Life-style Blue's haircut is that it make her look absolutely gorgeous—the cut and style should flatter her face, and the style should be manageable enough that she can leave her home each day looking as good as she did when she walked out of the beauty salon. She can probably wear her hair any length.

Short hair: The Blue woman should only choose short hair if it is the most flattering to her face and figure. She needn't pick a haircut because it's easy to care for, since her hairstylist should be able to show her how to manage any style of any length—after all, she has enough time in the morning to do anything her hair requires.

If she picks short hair, it should be layered for body, staying power, and softness. At all costs, the Life-style Blue woman should avoid plastering her hair with spray to make it hold until her next appointment. A little teasing, hot rollers, and a curling iron can make short hair into any number of flattering styles. The short cut should not be severe; a perm may not be necessary.

A short haircut does have to be maintained perfectly, and depending on how fast your hair grows, you may need a trim every three–four weeks. A Life-style Blue woman should not have trouble keeping a standing haircut appointment, so many short styles are available to her.

Medium-length hair: Medium-length hair may seem very boring to the Life-style Blue woman, who would probably rather have the versatility of longer hair or the reliability of shorter hair. But medium-length hair is a good safety point, because it is most flattering to almost everyone. For the woman who is considering making the transition from short to long hair, medium is a very good length to have while deciding. It gives a woman the benefit of softness from a lot of hair—and many faces need to be surrounded by hair—but doesn't cause the problem of too much hair. When in doubt, medium is always the best length.

Some Life-style Blues have a permanent, because this helps their hair keep its curl. But many of these women do not need one since they are so often at the beauty salon, their hairstylist is able to give them all the help they need. Since it is hard on the hair to combine a perm with a daily dose of electric rollers, the Life-style Blue can easily damage her hair, and she should try to avoid it.

Long hair: Long hair and Life-style Blues go well together, because long hair needs proper care to look its best, and Life-style Blues have the most time for themselves and their hair. Long hair should probably be cut with some layers, which should be carefully maintained by the hairstylist. No Life-style Blue ought to wear long straight hair. Darling, that would be a sin. The hair can be layered all over or cut in two parts so the top is layered and the bottom is long. For some people I cut the hair so it is almost one length, and then I do a lot of layers on the last two inches so the curl stays just right.

Long hair can be soft and stylish and sexy and should never be sprayed or worn in a severe style. You can put it up at night or pull back for sports if you need to. You can set a classic cut in many different ways—you have a world of versatility at your fingertips. Enjoy it, darling.

NIGHT LIFE

Because Life-style Blue women have the most time for their hair, they have the greatest number of choices when it comes to doing something a little different for an evening out. Many Blues choose to go to the hairdresser for special occasions, but you can do so many things with your hair that you may want to experiment with some of them before you book your next appointment. Or ask your hairstylist to try some of these techniques and then decide together how you like them.

• Pin curls. That's right, darling—old-fashioned pin curls, from the good old days. If you don't have a permanent and you are looking for a lot of curl, fluff, or fullness for one day or a special occasion, pin curls will give it to you. And it's hard to damage your hair with this simple method. Wet or spritz your hair and make small to medium-sized curls. You may want to use a setting lotion (or even stale beer) for the curls, to give your hair a little more body and holding power, but don't do this often, as excessive use of gels or lotions can dry your hair.

• Tissue-paper rollers. Before they had electric curlers or even wire rollers, women set their hair in rags (honestly). They tied the end of a strand of hair with a rag, rolled the strand to the scalp, and then tied the rag to secure the curl. If you don't happen to have a rag in your home that you're willing to put in your hair, try tissue paper or Kleenex or aluminum foil instead. The cost is minimal, and you toss the curler away when you are finished. Your hair will have a soft, wavy curl and suffer no damage from hot rollers.

• Put it up. Some people think that when they can't do anything else with their hair, they'll put it up, because that's safe. That's fine, but there are so many creative ways to do it, darling, that you should consider this method for nighttime. Even if you have medium-length hair—or if it's short but not too short—you can tie up a section of your hair and wrap it in gold cord or black velvet ribbon or twist a pearl necklace into it, and the result will be very dramatic. Putting your hair up should not make you look like a schoolmarm. Play around in front of your mirror with your collection of hair accessories and jewelry. See what you can do by braiding and putting the hair up, by braiding sections and leaving the rest of your hair down, by putting a ponytail a little off center, or by putting up the tendrils next to your face. Forget about severity and aim for a soft, sexy, and alluring look. Not all face shapes look good with the hair up, so experiment. There's usually something very creative you can do that will be right for the occasion and your face.

That's All Folks

When I first came to America, before I got a job, I would stay home and watch television some of the day to help my English get better. It was on American television that I first heard the expression "That's All Folks" from some cartoon character whose English was not any better than my own.

So this is the end of the book. It is not all folks, because hopefully as your hair grows and your life evolves you will use the book over and over again.

Please remember that the length of your hair has very little to do with your life-style. Cutting your hair from long to short will not make you change from a life-style blue to a life-style red. I am sure that the women in this book—and you too—will go through various stages during which you will want to try long, short, and medium-length hair. For many years, I have worked with actresses who wanted long, full hair. Now, as we get deeper into the 80's, I feel a trend toward shorter and lighter hair. Some of my clients will decide to cut. Others will decide to grow. Still others will wait and see. But change is constant; it is a part of everyone's life.

Whether you are a Life-style Red, Green, or Blue, as time goes by and fashions change, you will want to update your look. But each time you decide to make a change—remember me. And remember your life-style. If you work with us together, you will never make a change you regret.

Meanwhile, work with your chosen hairstylist and the pages of this book. Fill in all the sheets and questionnaires. Help me to help you. You are going to look the best you have ever looked in your life.

Then shake your head, darling.

Run your fingers through your glorious hair and smile.

Call or come by if you're ever in Beverly Hills. I want to see you in person if I can. And if you have any problems, don't forget to fill in an extra worksheet and send it to me with a picture. Au revoir, darling.

Jose Eber
Maurice/Jose
9426 Santa Monica Blvd.
Beverly Hills, California 90210

Are you a Life-style Red, like Farrah —ready for a swim or a set of tennis at the drop of a sun hat? Are you a Life-style Green, as Brenda Vaccaro is, with a world of business waiting for you to wing in and make the decisions? Or are you Life-style Blue, like Cher, with a special glamour you are ready and willing to spend time to perfect? You should know for sure— and so should your hairdresser.

This attention to life-style is Jose Eber's key to success—one of the major reasons celebrities clamor to have him do their hair. Now he and his celebrity clients share their secrets with you.

In *Shake Your Head, Darling* you find his beauty work sheets that help you identify your face shape, guidelines to help you identify your hair type, but, most important of all, quizzes that zero in on your life-style. Just as Jose does for the stars, he helps you find the real you so you can choose the right hairdo.

Treating you as he does his famous clients, Jose gives you the facts on hair conditioning and selecting the right length and color, and suggests a morning hair-care routine to fit your life. And, as they are in Jose's salon, the stars themselves are everywhere—photographed in their newest hairstyles, commenting on beauty basics, encouraging you to adopt the life-style approach that works for them and can work for you.